STO

ACPL ITEM
DISCARDED

ALLEN COUNTY PUBLIC LIBRARY

3 1833 00067

SO-BWS-203

JUL 27 '78

STAY YOUNG

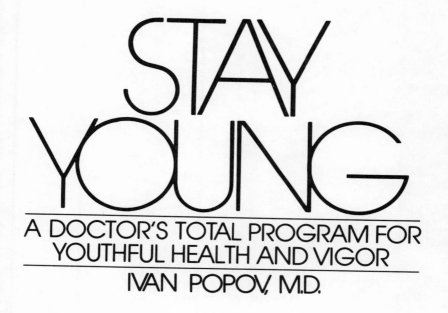

STAY YOUNG

A DOCTOR'S TOTAL PROGRAM FOR YOUTHFUL HEALTH AND VIGOR

IVAN POPOV, M.D.

GROSSET & DUNLAP
PUBLISHERS   NEW YORK

Copyright © 1975 by Ivan Popov, M.D.
All rights reserved
Published simultaneously in Canada

Library of Congress catalog card number: 73-22740
ISBN 0-448-11697-9

First Printing
Printed in the United States of America

2010572

To the memories of
Alexis Carrel, Axel Munthe, and Ranko Kovljanic,
whose philosophies
so influenced my way of thinking.

Contents

Part III: Revitalizing Techniques That Can Work

Part IV: The Science of Revitalization

Part V: A Revitalized You

Selected Readings 271

Index 281

Acknowledgments

This book is the result of decades of reading, researching, experimenting and observing. However I am especially indebted for the little knowledge I have acquired in revitalization to:

Charles BERNET, M.D. who made me understand the unlimited therapeutic possibilities of seawater;

Charles CARTOTTO, M.D., the sole famous surgeon I know of, who said that the best operation is the one not performed;

Emmanuel CHERASKIN, M.D., D.M.D., whose writing has made me appreciate the possibility of predictive medicine;

Elliott GOLDWAG, Ph.D. who made my dream of a multi-therapeutic clinic a reality, and his brother,

William GOLDWAG, M.D. whose considerable medical knowledge helped so much to start the clinic;

Professor Henri GRIFFON, Ph.D., the only real genius I have had the opportunity to meet;

René HENRY, M.D., the indefatigable fighter for the acceptance of new and just approaches in medicine;

Walter LORENZ, M.D., a clever old practitioner who makes working with him a daily pleasure;

Patrick McGRADY, Jr. whose writings helped the idea of revitalization to be accepted;

Jean MORELLE, Ph.D. who succeeded in solving many biochemical problems by following nature instead of competing with it;

Norman ORENTREICH, M.D. whose encyclopedic mind made me feel richer after each meeting with him;

Denis de ROUGEMONT whose writing and long conversations have helped me to understand many of the riddles of modern civilization;

Abraham SHAMES who explained to me in simple terms many complicated problems of American culture;

Professor Franz SCHMID, M.D. whose notable kindness with children is equalled only by his notable knowledge of cell-therapy;

Joachim STEIN, M.D., the learned cell-therapist and researcher;

Max WOLF, M.D., one of the oldest researchers in age, yet one of the youngest in mind, I have had the pleasure to know.

And in preparing the manuscript, I owe my greatest debt to Alexander Dorozynski, the former European editor of *Medical World News*, whose mastery of languages, vast knowledge of scientific and medical history and research, and brilliant writing made this book a reality.

A Note to the Reader

None of the procedures described in this book
should be undertaken
unless a physician has first been consulted
as to the condition sought to be treated
and the effect of the procedures intended to be used.

In preparing this material I have drawn from the research of many of my colleagues in science and medicine of both past and present, in addition to the experience of my own years of work and practice. If I have omitted anyone or misrepresented any findings it is most assuredly through oversight and not intent, and would welcome the opportunity to correct any such error in future printings.

Introduction

I have practiced medicine for 40 years. Nearly 30 of these I have devoted to revitalization. Revitalization is not a specialty that deals with a single system or function of the body, but with the treatment and prevention of a multitude of degenerative diseases that manifest themselves in the form of premature aging.

I have also engaged in research and have followed closely research carried out by other physicians and biologists. I have visited many countries either as a treating or consulting physician, or simply to learn of the research being conducted there. In the past few decades, I have witnessed extraordinary progress in pharmacology, genetics, endocrinology, surgery and other medical specialties. Advances made in the past 50 years can be compared to those made in the past 3,000 years.

And yet, there is something about all this that I cannot accept: man does not seem to benefit from these advances as much as he should. On the contrary, he seems to be growing older faster, often deprived of the joys of a full, active, prolonged lifespan.

In my opinion, the reasons are threefold: 1) Civilization has brought about stresses that even its own splendid medical advances cannot overcome; 2) The scattering of advanced medical research over the globe, and even within countries, is so great that it is not shared and sifted so that man can gain from it as rapidly as it is available; and 3) The combination of these two has encouraged both man and his doctors to forget that he is a whole — body, mind and spirit. Man has been separated, for scientific purposes, into a series of organs and syndromes. This is how he sees himself, and how the physicians and researchers see him when they work at cures. Not as a complete entity — a product of nature and not of science — whose whole organism can be affected, and should be so treated, when part of it breaks down.

It is even more disturbing that man has accepted this as a normal state of affairs, although there seems to be a gradual increase in awareness of the problem and desire to change it. (I hope, with this book, to help with those changes.) He appears resigned to the accumulation in his body of ever-growing ailments. In his 50's, in his 40's, and increasingly in his 30's, he begins to acquire degenerative diseases said to be "on the subclinical level." The symptoms are too vague for the disease to be treated or identified, but it is there; it has not been *prevented*. Then when it is too late, he comes to accept as his normal lot emphysema, heart disease, overweight, depression, fatigue, loss of energy and sexual powers and enjoyment. He does not use the means at his disposal to prevent this. His vitality is eroded, first gradually and then more quickly. He has aged prematurely.

This strikes me as nothing short of scandalous, because it need not happen. I am not a licensed physician in America, but I have treated many, many American patients over the years. Even in that most advanced country in the world, man does not enjoy the longest — or the healthiest — lifespan among nations. In fact, the average lifespan in America seems to be getting shorter, as it is in many industrialized countries.

I think that everybody is entitled to live the fullest possible life that modern science can help achieve. I have had patients who in their 80's and 90's retained vigorous mental and physical powers, led creative lives, and enjoyed good food and active sex lives. They did not give in to premature aging, and neither should you. Premature aging deprives you of good years of life, or transforms these years into a burden — for yourself and others. If you'd strike for better wages, you should strike for better health. You have a right to it. And there are things that can be done.

You may not be able to change, from one day to the next, the life you lead, or the environment to which you are subjected. But there are many small choices you can make that taken together can help you prevent premature aging.

Aging manifests itself in many ways. I have read many books, most of them written by doctors, that tell you how to exercise against heart disease, how to have a better sex life, how to stop smoking, or how to lose weight. I have found that none approach man as a whole, body and spirit — these two are inseparable and interact upon each other. None of them put at your disposal the synthesis of knowledge and experience that makes it possible to prevent, or at least retard, the array of wasting diseases that represent premature loss of vitality.

We know that modern pharmacology has taken giant steps, providing mankind with powerful, effective drugs. But at the same time, it has relegated to oblivion the many traditional remedies made not by corporations, but by nature. I have seen how much the measured use of natural remedies can achieve. They should not be overlooked, but should be brought out of oblivion.

And finally, I have practiced in, founded, or directed several revitalization centers — places whose purpose is to treat the conditions of aging — and have had the opportunity to see the results that can be achieved. A combination of therapies, taken from both science and nature and directed at the whole man, not just a part of him, can produce remarkable benefits.

There are revitalization centers in most countries of the world, but they are reserved for a privileged few, because such treatments are costly. I do not think the benefits of such modern revitalization methods should be restricted to an elite of political, financial, or other leaders, or to those (such as actors or doctors) who are particularly conscious of the problems of aging and who take the trouble to find out what can be done about it.

Some of the things I have to say are simple, commonsense observations, the result of many years of practice. Others are the conclusions of exhaustive research. Some may be well known and widely accepted; others, such as cell therapy, are not only controversial, they are not even permitted in some countries, including the United States. However, this book is not a crusade to change the world. It is not a book to diagnose your trouble and prescribe your cure — there can be no such book, unless it is directed only at you and is printed in a single copy.

On the whole, the book is intended to let you know what can be done to live not only longer, but better and more fully, in the world that exists. A world that is overcrowded, where pesticides are used and will continue to be used, where available food is either in short supply or short in quality.

It is not a book on sexual behavior, although the subject will be dealt with, not a book on nutrition — I have yet to see one succeeding in the impossible task of suiting everybody — not a book on stress, although I believe stress to be the number one enemy of our time. Our ancestors were occasionally subjected to stress, and it was not without value, because if it didn't kill them, it gave strength to their adaptive potential. In our society, minor stresses are constantly gnawing.

The book does not claim to give you the one answer, but a lot of small answers. Life is a list of countless choices, and I hope to help you make some of them. Not by instructing you, dogmatically, in what to do, but by trying to explain some of the background so you can make the decisions.

And it doesn't matter how insignificant each decision seems to be: a choice between a steak and a TV dinner, between a bottle of soda pop and a glass of water, between a book and a TV special, a walk and a ride, a potato chip and a bean sprout. The important thing is that they add up to a healthier, fuller, better life.

It would be foolish to suggest that I know all the answers or to pretend I am always right. This book is the result of a lifetime of concern for the preservation of health, but also a book reflecting my own human frailties and personal biases. For instance, I have come to rely increasingly on remedies provided by nature. I am hardly a faddist. It is simply one of the many solutions reached in my experience. Such biases as this are unavoidable when dealing with life — because life is always too vast to fit into *any* formula.

Part I:
What
Civilization
Is Doing to Us

1. Living vs. Merely Surviving

Twentieth-century civilization has brought us many extraordinary things: airplanes that will take us anywhere in the world on a moment's notice; freedom from the ravages of disease; relief from many of the daily chores of the past. It has given us motion pictures on tables, boxes we can carry around to tell us what is happening in the world and sometimes even in the universe.

It has taught us to dispose of outworn objects, and it has always provided new and better ones in their places. The advancements in almost every area of science have yielded exciting changes in the way we live, and the advancements seem to be hurtling forward at an almost unstoppable pace. It seems there will always be something newer, something more complete, something better. We have learned to rely on science to solve our problems for us.

But there is one flaw: science has not taught us how to replace ourselves when *we* wear out. It is true that we have an average longevity much greater than that of our tribal ancestors who were deprived of our vaccinations, antibiotics, obstetricians, organ transplants, psychotherapists, and gerontologists (those who study the process of aging). But we seem to age faster.

Some striking figures prove this. In 1972 the World Health Organization issued its statistical report in which epidemiologists and computer specialists calculated for 34 countries both the life expectancy at birth and the life expectancy for persons who had already reached 65. What made the report significant was not its evidence that those countries with high life expectancies at birth were the industrial nations where medicine had overcome the plagues of childhood. Instead, it was the news that a man's life expectancy at 65 was greater in Greece (79.3 years) and Iceland (80.3 years), two of the least industrialized nations in the world, than it was in the United States (77.8 years). In fact, 23 of the 34 nations reporting showed a drop in the life expectancy of their 65-year-olds from the previously recorded 1958 figures. With the single exception of Japan, all the highly industrialized nations were in this group of 23.

These figures are not widely known, and people who learn of them usually accept them without asking questions. Yet, they mean that if you are 50 or 60 years old, and live in the United States, your life expectancy is lower than it was for someone your age only 10 or 20 years ago. This is shocking in a world where we are transplanting kidneys and hearts, and from which we can fly to the moon.

Even more disturbing is the increase in degenerative, or wasting, diseases such as hypertension, cardiovascular ailments, emphysema — diseases that turn us from people into patients long before our time. Another computation from the same agency dramatically illustrates this. In the United States, the elimination of cardiovascular diseases alone would increase life expectancy at birth by something over 12 years for men, and 10 for women. These are extraordinary figures. The elimination of a single category of diseases, even granting that it is the most important one, would increase an American man's expected lifespan at birth from 66.6 years to 79, and a woman's from 74 to 84!

Clearly, what we've gained on one side, we're losing on the other. Though modern medicine has protected us from many diseases that were lethal in the past, it has failed to protect us from premature aging. Why?

The Failure of Modern Medicine

Medicine, not unlike physics, has undergone a phase of intensive specialization, and in both fields this has led to an awkward situation. Physicists have discovered dozens of subatomic particles of matter and antimatter, each with disconcerting properties. Having taken the atom apart, they don't quite know how to put it together again. There is no unified theory that can account for everything that is known about matter and energy, and the mass of observations that have been made often appears to be in conflict.

Physicists have become specialists in low-energy physics, or high-energy particles, or relativity, or astrophysics. Physicians have become neurologists, neurosurgeons, endocrinologists, cancerologists, or gastroenterologists. In pursuing intensive specialization, they have lost sight of man as a whole. What has happened is a dehumanization of medicine.

This dehumanization has resulted from the shortage of "primary doctors," a shortage that has become increasingly severe. Thirty or 40 years ago, approximately 70 percent of the graduating medical doctors in the United States became general practitioners; the others turned to various specialties. As the public became conditioned to think that specialists knew better, the doctors discovered that specialties brought academic recognition, higher income, and social prestige. A specialist became "somebody special," and a shift so drastic was made that by a few years ago the ratio had been reversed: some 70 percent of graduating physicians turned to specialties, and only 30 percent or so became general practitioners.

At the same time, a cleavage developed between doctors of different "schools." This became particularly apparent in the different ways medicine was practiced from country to country. If anything should be international, medicine should, yet as medical science progressed, the difference in medical practices increased from one country to another.

There is a general impression in the United States that European medicine is somewhat backward, and, in turn, there is a feeling in Europe that American medicine is mechanistic. Where is the truth? Almost all Americans accept as a matter of course that American medicine is the best in the world. Yet Americans receive far from the best medical care, health and longevity in the United States compare rather unfavorably with health and longevity in some other countries, and infant mortality in America is far from being the world's lowest.

There is no doubt in my mind that the answer lies somewhere between the two assumptions. We have a right to be proud of the achievements of medicine, but we haven't won *all* the battles yet.

Overspecialization vs. the Holistic Approach

Knowledge has accumulated so rapidly since the beginning of the century that superspecialization was unavoidable. It has made it possible to develop some extremely refined techniques for the diagnosis, treatment, and prevention of many diseases. But at the same time as the science of medicine developed, some of the art of medicine was forgotten. A sort of imaginary world was created, inhabited not by men and women, but by disembodied symptoms, syndromes, and diseases described in medical textbooks. The successes achieved have been heady, but we have lost our humility. We must recognize that what we know is infinitely smaller than what we don't know.

The answers that science has provided to some of our questions have led to a belief that a scientific explanation is required by, and can be made to account for, every empirical observation. If the laboratories could not come forth with such an explanation, it became simpler to reject the unexplained phenomenon altogether.

The result has been, on the one hand, highly refined techniques based on the analysis of some sophisticated "organic mechanisms," and on the other hand, a narrowed view that does not encompass man as a whole.

I have always viewed man as a body-mind unit that cannot be entirely explained in terms of biochemistry, physiology, pharmacology, and physics. The emphasis on only one form of rational scientific thought has led to a disregard of one of man's most important attributes, that of intuition — an educated kind of intuitive feeling has always been a fundamental part of medical art. The vagueness of the term "feeling" is in itself unacceptable to science, yet it is at the basis of any art, including the art of medicine.

This feeling is not easy to define, yet it has contributed to the greatness of clinical medicine in the western world. It involves the use of the eyes, the ears, the senses of touch, smell, and taste as well as the human experience of the physician making a diagnosis. It works in association with scientific knowledge. It is, in my opinion, a prerequisite to the making of a great clinician. I consider myself fortunate to have had the opportunity to study and work with such physicians.

As a youth, I spent a year as an intern in a hospital in Paris. I clearly remember the first day, when I and half a dozen other aspiring practitioners were introduced into the general medicine department headed by a Professor Sergent. We expected a masterly discourse, but instead we were taken into a ward filled with patients and told to remain silent and observe: to sit, watch, listen, and smell. An hour or so later, Professor Sergent took us to another ward, and gave us the same instructions. We had never seen any of the patients before, nor did we know what diseases they were suffering from. In the afternoon, the same lesson was repeated in a third ward, but before it began the Professor told us that the patients in the first ward had been suffering from lung cancer and those in the second ward from lung tuberculosis. The patients in the third ward were suffering from either lung cancer or tuberculosis, and we were again asked to watch, listen, and smell and then try to tell which of the two diseases each patient had. Interestingly enough, the simple diagnosis made by completely inexperienced youngsters, without the help of any laboratory tests or microscopic examinations, proved to be accurate in well over half the cases.

Later, of course, we learned advanced medical and biological techniques which added to our diagnostic and therapeutic capabilities, but these techniques also detracted from the more all-encompassing, or holistic, approach to man. Patients were shared by specialists, fragmented, and increasingly isolated from the human contact that is so essential a part of treatment.

We also became separated from our patients, not only by desks, nurses, and assistants, but by equipment.

Fortunately, doctors have now come to recognize the shortcomings of overspecialization, and have started a new trend toward holistic medicine — a concern not only with the parts man is made of, but with the entire mind-body unit. There is still much reform needed but there have been a number of encouraging signs. For instance, a few years ago the American Board of Family Practice was created to function on the same level as other "specialty" boards. It is ironic, in a way, that family practice is now classified as a specialty, but it is also understandable. It corresponds to the elevated public image of the specialist, and also recognizes the fact that general practice requires certification and recertification (every seven years) on the basis of an examination and a review of the work of the physician requesting it.

In the past few years, more young doctors have been turning to general or family practice, and the earlier trend is gradually reversing. These family doctors are more than ever aware of the fantastic progress that has been made in the medical specialties, and they know how much this progress can increase the efficacy of holistic medicine.

Moreover, there is a trend toward the recognition and the use of facts that are empirically known but not scientifically explained. The lofty world of science has rediscovered humility, and this is a good thing, for as doctors we cannot afford to ignore anything that can benefit our patients — whether it is a chemical formula or not.

Thus acupuncture — considered yesterday as not much more than an entertaining bit of Oriental folklore — is now studied and practiced in the most respectable hospitals and medical centers in the western world.

Likewise, unexplained psychic phenomena — until only a few years ago relegated to the world of superstition and myth, and studied by few scientists (generally regarded as oddballs) — are now not only studied, but used in the practice of medicine.

These phenomena can pave the way to an entirely new kind of medicine, putting to use the power of the mind in the treatment and prevention of organic diseases. Physicians of renown have started speaking of yoga and of the ancient Vedic traditions of India. Yet why should we be surprised by the power of the brain — billions of interacting cells that represent about 2 percent of the body's weight, and 10 percent of its metabolic processes?

It has been discovered that a variety of diseases can be "mind treated," with the use of biofeedback training. Considering that the term "biofeedback" was coined only in 1969, the progress that has been made in the field is amazing. It is no longer a laboratory wonder, but a therapeutic tool that has been successfully applied to some of the most stubborn diseases of civilization. We will examine biofeedback at greater length in Chapter 16.

These advances notwithstanding, it is still a commonplace that today's doctor often doesn't even touch his patient, who, uneasy, dissatisfied, may keep coming back to find the human, compassionate relationship so essential to medicine. He keeps coming back, but he does not find what he needs. The consequences are unfortunate, but only recently have we started to recognize them and try to do something about them.

One result of depersonalized medicine is the abusive use of drugs. The unsatisfied patient who keeps returning to his doctor with vague complaints is labeled a hypochondriac, a neurotic bothered by vague symptoms of unknown origin. The physician finds this relationship frustrating, and tends to justify his role in it by writing a prescription to avoid having the patient — and himself — grow even more dissatisfied and uneasy. The prescribed drug is frequently aimed at the symptoms of an organic disease, because the flaw in the body mechanism that has led to the disease is itself overlooked. It can only be discovered through the deep involvement of the physician with his patient as a whole. Meanwhile, a pain-relieving drug may be prescribed against chest pain, a tranquilizer against sleeplessness.

The "nuisance patient" wouldn't be one if he didn't have some problem. But since he cannot really confide in his doctor, and may hesitate to turn to his priest or minister, he is isolated, and doesn't have much of a chance. Psychotropic drugs may mask his problem, but they will increase his dependency and instability. If psychotropic drugs don't do the trick, he may be referred to a psychiatrist. This can be compared to killing flies with an elephant gun.

The diagnosis of these patients should dig much deeper. Many dissatisfactions in life are translated into symptoms. The cause is forgotten, and man ends up living permanently on pills. Vitality leaks out through the cracks, and the organism yields to degenerative diseases characteristic of premature aging.

How Long a Life Can We Expect?

The question of premature aging always raises another one: how long should we reasonably expect to live? Does nature have a clock for us? When would it naturally stop without disease or accidents interfering? Zoologists are not unanimous about the lifespans of animals. It is believed that the tortoise lives up to 150 or 200 years; the vulture, 120; the Indian elephant, 60 to 70; the hippopotamus, the rhinoceros, and some whales, 50; the chimpanzee, 30 to 40; the lion, the pigeon, and the frog, 30 to 35; the rabbit, 12; the sparrow, 9; and the lowly ant, up to 20.

When it comes to man, let us disregard legendary longevity, such as Methuselah's 969 years, which were more likely lunar years (or months), making the patriarchal lifespan slightly over 80 years.

Gerontologists are intrigued by the existence of a few pockets of exceptional longevity on the globe. In recent years, serious studies have confirmed that people have lived up to 130 and 140 years and even, in one case, above 150. Such longevity is exceptional not only for the age itself, but for the retained vigor, continued activity, and zest not usually associated with senility.

Dr. Alexander Leaf, chief of medical services at Massachusetts General Hospital, and professor at the Harvard University Medical School, reported the results of a two-year study financed by the National Geographic Society in the January 1973 issue of *National Geographic* magazine. He visited three such Shangri-Las: the region of Abkhazia, located in the Caucasus mountains above the Black Sea in the Georgian Soviet Socialist Republic; the land of the Hunza in the Karakoram range in Kashmir; and the Andean valley of Vilcabamba, in Ecuador.

The 1970 census of the Caucasus region listed 1,884 centenarians in the Georgian SSR — 39 per 100,000 population. There were 2,500 centenarians in neighboring Azerbaijan SSR — 63 per 100,000. This makes this region's proportion of centenarians some 20 times higher than it is in the United States. The oldest living man in the area was Shiraly Mislimov, of Azerbaijan, said to have been born in 1805. He died in 1974.

Dr. Leaf did not meet Mislimov, but during his journey he made many physical examinations and talked to many centenarians — the oldest being "a sprightly lady named Khfaf Lasuria." Dr. Leaf writes that "She had a lot to tell because her memory was good — and she was more than 130 years old."

In Hunza, the dating problem was more difficult because there are no written records. There also seemed to be, however, an unusually large number of centenarians, and the oldest Hunzukut was said to be 110 years old.

In Vilcabamba, where the population is of Spanish descent, there are written baptismal records. The two oldest men there were 123 and 142 years old.

But far more important than the precise chronological age are the reasons why, in these three regions, so many vigorous, lively old people are found. Are they exceptions because there are some unknown factors that turn their villages into "life preserves," or are these regions representative of man's *real* longevity potential, a potential that is eroded in the rest of the world by factors that accelerate the aging process?

All of these exceptionally old people, or nearly all, are active, alert and healthy, as if past a certain point they grew no older. Dr. David Davies, a gerontologist at University College in London, who also visited the Vilcabamba valley, reported in *New Scientist* that the unusually old inhabitants he saw "seemed as bright, alert, and upright, with excellent dental health, as those several decades younger. . . . All seemed to be going about simple tasks, such as hoeing, which were yet of benefit to the community." There is no such thing as retirement. Centenarians continue to play a useful role in the community.

Dr. Leaf, who was in his early 50's and quite fit, sometimes found it difficult to keep up with the centenarians he was interviewing. One man, who claimed to be 106 years old, had climbed up a muddy, slippery, and steep incline to spend the summer with his herd of goats. It took Dr. Leaf six hours to catch up with him. He writes: "My own elation over getting up to the pasture lands was quelled when I was informed that the old man made the same trek in just half of the time it had taken me." On another occasion, Dr. Leaf was exhausted when he followed a 117-year-old man who had carried a pail of potatoes up a hill.

Another point common to the three regions is that old people did not eat much. The average daily caloric intake was around 1,900, while in America, the average for all ages is estimated to be over 3,000 calories. This fits with research carried out many years ago by Dr. Clive McCay, nutritionist at Cornell University. Dr. McCay showed that rats, underfed but given all the vitamins and trace elements they required, had a lifespan increased by about 30 percent. This fits also, of course, with the knowledge that overreating and obesity radically reduce longevity.

Yet Dr. Davies noted with surprise that in Vilcabamba people drank two to four cups of rum a day, and smoked from 40 to 60 homemade cigarettes. Dr. Leaf states that he was amazed at the amounts of vodka, brandy, and wine drunk in Abkhazia and

Georgia, at least on festive occasions. He even came upon obese centenarians, "a phenomenon I would have not thought possible."

The Lessons of the Centenarians

It seems that many of these exceptionally old people remained sexually active well into their 80's and 90's. They usually shied away from speaking about their sex lives, so this point has never been clearly established.

In my experience, I have found that sexual activity is a normal function which, in a healthy man, lasts as long as life itself. A happy love life and a healthy sex life undoubtedly contribute to longevity. This is also true, of course, with regard to women. In women, hormone therapy can be a useful part of the multitherapeutic approach to revitalization and, started at the appropriate time, can postpone menopause by 10 and even 20 years.

Most of the people I have treated are sexually active, no matter what their age. Not long ago, a known figure in the world of arts, whom I had treated for nearly 20 years, suddenly died. He was over 90. A few days after his death, I received a letter from his regular physician, who wrote: "He died a natural death . . . not of degenerative disease, and working with as much gusto and creativity as ever." And on the eve of his death he had boasted to this physician of having had a very pleasant interlude with a girl almost 70 years his junior.

A common point was observed among the people who live an exceptionally long life: nearly all of them were married. Dr. Leaf notes that Professor G. E. Pitzkhelauri, director of the gerontological center in Tbilisi in the Georgian SSR, has studied thousands of records of old people, and has found that *only* those who are married live to be exceptionally old. Some couples have been married for more than 100 years! Mislimov, the 168-year-old veteran of them all, claimed to have been married for 102 years. He was 65 when he took an 18-year-old bride; she was still alive, at age 120, in 1973.

Another feature common to all of the longevity pockets is that old people are not rejected by society, but, quite the contrary, have an important status, occupy a privileged position, and are respected for their wisdom. Retirement from active life, rejection by society, and the feeling of being a burden are introductions to death. A recent experience in Israel makes the point. A group of old people, instead of being placed in retirement homes, were given a shoemaking plant to operate. The business prospered, and so did the old people, who soon started accepting "youngsters" in their 60's.

Your own attitude toward aging is also important. In Abkhazia as well as in Georgia, people *expect* to live to be 100 or more; centenarians remember their 80's as still being part of youth.

And, of course, they are healthy. Degenerative diseases, so characteristic of industrial society, are very rare. Dr. Davies notes that in Vilcabamba, "accidents, or diseases brought from outside the area, were the usual cause of death."

There are other regions where people live particularly long and active lives: in the Siberian tundras, in the Balkans, in Central and South America, in the Himalayan mountains. Even in our industrial society, some people live well into their 100's. Why?

None of the investigators who have tackled the question have come up with a single answer. But there are several recurrent themes: pure air, pure water, usually rather cool climates, natural and not overly abundant food, continued sexual activity, and work. And, above all, the joy of being alive.

"Every day is a gift when you are over a hundred," a Georgian farmer, who had celebrated his 100th anniversary a few weeks earlier, told Dr. Leaf.

Old age — or, rather, prolonged youth — is in the mind as well as in the body.

2. The Multitherapeutic Approach to Staying Young

The first thing to understand about premature aging is that there is actually no specific disease of aging. Instead, somewhere along the line, one or more of the parts begins to break down, and it is when this breakdown is sufficiently advanced that we see the signs of the related disease. Only then do science and formal medicine enter the picture, to repair or halt the damage.

When we talk about revitalization, or combating premature aging, we do not mean making people younger. We cannot turn the clock back — why should we want to? With maturity come many of the most exciting blessings of life, such as wisdom, understanding, and tolerance. We mean preserving the whole organism — body and mind — of man in good and vigorous health for as long as nature intended.

Doing this is a form of preventive medicine, but it does not come in a package. It is not like a vaccination you might take against polio or smallpox (you cannot take a vaccination against time). It is not something you can only do up to a certain point, after which it is too late. It is rather a matter of understanding yourself, and of using the lessons of nature and of science to help preserve and maintain your powers at prime functioning level. Whether this is for the enjoyment of your work, of your sex life, of your family, of your leisure time, it can only benefit you.

During the four decades I have been practicing medicine I have witnessed the increasing incidence of diseases and accelerated aging processes that are directly the result of the environment we have created and the way of life that goes with it. In dealing with this, I am not advocating that we step backwards, nor am I rejecting scientific and technical progress. But we should not forget our bond with nature. Nature does not cheat, but everybody cheating nature pays a heavy penalty.

I know that it is within your potential to change your life, if you only reject some of the false premises we have foisted upon ourselves, because we have been caught in the whirlpool that we have created.

Unfortunately, it is easy to give in to the temptations of our situation. Never before has man possessed so many material means that should give him time to develop his personality, self-expression, health and well-being, and a life that needn't be cut short by illness, nor end up in years of humiliating, aimless senility. And yet, because of our material means, we have been too busy to remember that there is something that we should not give up, something that doesn't require our giving up anything else we already have.

I am talking about vitality. The key to staying young is not cosmetics, or plastic surgery, or hair dye or massive doses of vitamins or chemical substances. For all the applications of technology can not keep us younger. All the compliments and admiring comments about active oldsters always seem to revolve around their energy and vitality. The "bloom of youth" is an impression not only of glowing skin and shining hair, but one of energy and joy in living. This can be sustained, and both in physical and mental terms can, and should be, encouraged and aided to continue into vigorous later years. That is the point of revitalization.

Probably the most important message I can bring you is that there does not seem to be one single magic bullet that can be aimed at the problem of aging. Seeking one has often led us astray down this or that path of this or that wonder panacea.

On the contrary, man is a complex combination of so many factors that we must always take the whole into account when we are dealing with any of the parts. Man is not only a kidney, a liver, a brain — he is a whole body, and he is not only body but also mind and spirit. A diseased mind can interrupt the life of a healthy body in many ways, and likewise a healthy mind can be destroyed by corporal diseases. At the basis of this destruction there could be a single, apparently trivial factor such as a shortage of vitamin C, which could ultimately cause death from scurvy, or low blood sugar, which could lead to mental illness.

Because of this multiplicity of factors, I think there will never be such a single bullet. The shotgun, or more scientifically, the multitherapeutic approach, is the one that I find must be used. Such an approach must always begin with a careful study of the individual in all his aspects. Once this has been accomplished, it can be decided which combination of therapies should be administered to treat, or revitalize, the person. The spectrum of therapies which I use can encompass natural remedies such as sea water baths and herbal teas, as well as the modern techniques of hormone and cell injections.

The point is not to reject any proven therapies that work, nor to apply one favored technique to the exclusion of others. The point is to revitalize the whole man, using all the means at our disposal.

2010572

Development of the Multitherapeutic Approach

I have come to my conclusions about the multitherapeutic approach, and the testing and selection of the variety of therapies involved, over many years. I have always, it seems, been bringing together the seeming dualities of practice and research, science and nature, body and spirit in my medical efforts. The two greatest influences in my medical life, who together formed the basis for this attitude, also seem widely apart at first glance. One was Alexis Carrel, a brilliant scientist and Nobel Laureate. The other was Ranko Kovljanic, a simple country doctor practicing in the mountains of Yugoslavia (whom in the future I shall refer to just as Ranko). The multitherapeutic approach was essentially inspired by them.

Surgery was my first medical specialty, and I had already practiced for a few years when I realized it did not satisfy me. It was productive and healing, but it did not give answers. I took up pharmacology and research, and came across Alexis Carrel's extraordinary *Man the Unknown*, a book which changed my life. Carrel advanced the theory that man was indeed more than the sum of his parts, and that he was a machine more splendid than anything we could imagine, or that science could create. He said that diagnostic techniques tended to treat man not as an entity to be preserved and protected, but instead waited for parts of the machine to break down and then attempted to fix them.

Carrel, a famous medical scientist whose research I discuss later in this volume, spent a lifetime trying to discover the elusive factor which lay at the root of the functioning of the organism: the enigma which has been called the youth factor. I, too, became fascinated with the exciting, almost detective-story aspect of this research. If we could only identify what it was we should preserve within ourselves in order to stay young and vigorous, we would have the answer. If we could no longer manufacture it, perhaps we could find it elsewhere in nature, or duplicate it in the laboratory.

Although research fascinated me, I was still a practicing doctor. Just as Carrel and his work had taught me the value and excitement of scientific research, Ranko, the other influence, taught me about medicine as a healing art. He also taught me that we should reject nothing, whether it came from the laboratory or from the garden, from the field or the forest, if it could help to heal us.

I first met Ranko when I was about 21 years old. He was an invalid — his back had been broken many years earlier when he saved a young girl from drowning — and he had been in a wheelchair ever since. He was an old friend of my father's, but I had never met him. His practice was at the famous Yugoslav spa of Vrnjci, near where I took a holiday when I was in medical school. My father asked me to look him up while I was there, but I was much too busy having fun to get around to it. Then I had a bad riding accident and was taken, unconscious, to the nearest doctor. When I came to, the doctor was at my side, feeling for broken bones or sprains. It was Ranko, and we became friends immediately.

Ranko truly had the most remarkable mental outlook and joyful spirit of any person I have ever encountered. I had not suffered badly in the fall, and spent the rest of my convalescence and holiday with him. As I watched him go about his seemingly impossible daily rounds I realized what an extraordinary fellow he was. It is possible that his physical affliction had sensitized his mind and hands beyond those of the rest of us. However, as one who was still in college, and learning every day the new advances of science which I would presumably be applying to my own patients, I was surprised to see how Ranko made use of various plants, herbs, teas, poultices, and the like in his treatments — especially because I knew in fact he was a distinguished man of science himself.

Part of this was because Ranko practiced at a spa, and perhaps this is a good time to explain how the spa, so long a tradition in European life, works. Spas are simply towns situated at natural mineral springs, where people take what amount to "health holidays." When they arrive they are not put in the care of a social director who organizes their activities, but in the care of a doctor. Frequently they are sent by their doctors at home, and bring their medical histories with them. The spa physician gives them an examination and prescribes dosages of the waters along with diet and sleep regimens.

Vrnjci, like many spas, had palatial accommodations for wealthy city visitors, but rested in a rural hamlet where the year-round residents were poor. During his fulltime schedule,

Ranko treated wealthy patients, and in what for anyone else would have been free time, he took care of the local peasantry. Often they had nothing more than a few eggs or a chicken with which to pay him. They could not afford the elaborate drugs or other advanced treatments which were dispensed at the spa, and they were often unable to describe their ailments in any but the crudest terms. And they never went to the doctor except in the direst situations. Most of the time they cured themselves, using folk practices which had been handed down from generation to generation. They were tough, hardy, and knowledgeable about staying strong and healthy. Their lives depended on it, since they worked the land.

Ranko explained to me that there is much in nature that we do not know, but much that we do know and we should use it. He taught me that rather than trying to bring the drugs of civilization to the peasants, he was delighted to have his practice amongst the farmers because he could bring their cures to civilization. He also learned from treating his local patients that, by listening to them, touching them, or learning that they might be suffering grief or anger, he was much better able to treat and prescribe for them than for his city patients, whom he saw only briefly. He also trusted his intuition — he had to rely on it more, perhaps, than people who could get around better — and his powers of deduction were very sharp.

Whenever it was possible I went back to visit this remarkable man. Adversity seemed to bedevil him, and yet he never gave in to it. You can imagine how impressive this was to a young, vigorous 21-year-old who had always had everything. Now that I am much older, and am far from having everything, I remain impressed.

I have continued to draw from the ideas of Carrel and Ranko in my development of therapies, and in combining them to help retard aging and revitalize the organism.

The hints and information given in this book are for you to draw from. Although I cannot diagnose for you I can encourage you to recognize your situation and recognize that you can change it to sustain, or even regain, vitality and retard the aging process.

The first stage is essentially a mental undertaking. Revitalizing your lifestyle means taking a good look at the way you live; seeing it clearly, and possibly changing your mind about a few things, and then changing those things. Whether you decide to increase your sexual activity or decrease your food intake — it can only be decided by you.

The next stage is looking through the series of small changes and choices available to you in your everday life — using sea water instead of table salt to get your full complement of trace elements, learning to better eliminate toxic wastes and so on.

And finally there is a description of the science and research of revitalization, the detective story which has stretched down over the past centuries and an explanation of embryotherapy and cell therapy — two revitalization therapies which I have researched and used extensively, and which are in wide application in many countries of the world.

All this will, I hope, result in a revitalized you.

Part II: Revitalizing Your Lifestyle

3. Stress and How to Conquer It

Now that we have seen how the simple but vigorous centenarians of Dr. Leaf's studies lived, let us see how our lives compare. This can start us on the road to "curing" our own premature aging before it starts.

To begin with, take a fresh look at the world around you. I mean a fresh look. Imagine that you are from a primitive civilization, or a time-traveler crossing a few centuries to visit the modern world. You land, for example, in a suburban New York community.

There are many strange things to wonder at — machines that freeze, machines that heat, machines that roll, machines that wash, machines that fly. A great many machines, and you should give yourself some time to admire them.

Then begin observing the quaint local customs, starting in the early hours of the morning when the suburban aborigine, instead of coming awake gently to the sun, is brutally jarred out of bed by an ear-splitting noise and swallows strange solids, liquids, and occasionally assorted chemicals packed in colorful capsules, before joining other natives in a twice-daily ritual which takes place in a noisy, uncomfortable, crowded, smelly, sometimes subterranean vehicle.

You will notice scores of such strange self-punishing customs, which can be associated with a number of diseases unknown in your world: colitis, gastric ulcer, gout, rheumatism, gallstones, asthma, emphysema, chronic respiratory diseases, frequent indigestion and constipation, hypertension, arteriosclerosis, and heart disease.

When I walk in the streets of New York, I feel like such an alien. I see people hustling, preoccupied, worried, seldom smiling or looking happy. On the coldest day I see some perspiring nervously, and on the hottest, some of the hands I shake are cold. People sit motionless behind desks hour after hour, yet they find this inactivity so fatiguing that it is difficult for them to make a simple decision. They are worn out even when they wake up, and exhausted again at five o'clock, when they need a drink or two to pick them up. They become so accustomed to fatigue they don't even notice it. Then one day when perchance they are not fatigued, they realize what they have been missing.

I hear people say they cannot sleep without a pill or come awake without another. I have spoken to people who can no longer have sexual enjoyment, although they should be perfectly functional; people who have sudden losses of memory and who misplace things; people so surrounded with material goods they shouldn't worry about them, yet who worry because they have to maintain their status, because they have to meet often imaginary commitments; people who are basically healthy or could easily be, but who are preoccupied with diseases, pounds, and calories, and whose cluttered medicine cabinets are miniature pharmacies; people who rush through a martini lunch, who are late home for dinner, who sacrifice their very lives to the golden calf, to their position, their ambition, their status — as others see it.

Civilized man is subject to more and a greater variety of diseases than is any other animal or any man living closer to nature, even in primitive conditions where there is little concern for hygiene.

While medical progress has succeeded in eliminating the great plagues of humanity (the last remaining widespread and potentially lethal infectious disease is influenza), the stresses imposed by modern society have eroded health and exposed man to an increasing number of degenerative, chronic diseases, unknown, or very rare, in more primitive societies.

Stress, Hormones, and the Abuse of Our Adaptive Potential

In the 1930's, Dr. Hans Selye, director of the Institute of Experimental Medicine and Surgery at the University of Montreal, started experiments that led to the development of a revolutionary concept: stress as a cause of disease and premature aging.

Dr. Selye, who has written many articles and books (notably *The Stress of Life*), has said that "essentially, stress is the consequence of the rate of wear and tear in a biologic system; the 'system' may be the organism as a whole . . . or one of its parts. . . ." Further, that stress accompanies any vital activity and, in a sense, parallels the intensity of life. It is increased during nervous tension, physical injury, infections, muscular work or any other strenuous activity.

Dr. Selye substantiated his theory with many experiments and with the study of the organism's hormonal secretions during stress. He concluded that the body defends itself against stress by increasing the secretion by the pituitary gland of the adrenocorticotrophic hormone (ACTH), which in turn stimulates the adrenal cortex (at the upper part of the kidneys) to produce corticoid hormones.

He maintained that each man is born with a certain amount of this adaptive energy or vitality, which is gradually used up by stress, so that true physiologic aging is not determined by the time elapsed since birth but by the total amount of drain on this vital supply.

In our society, stress is *the* single most important factor of aging and ill health. Fortunately, not only can we reduce stress, but we can also restore our dwindling supply of adaptive energy. This is done through revitalization, and that's what this book is about.

If man is a machine, he is a self-repairing one. Given a chance, his body repairs not only parts of itself but the whole. I have never seen a man who has died of old age, and I don't think there is such a thing. (Of course, at some point, something must give.) People die because the weakest link in the human machine gives way. The weakest link is either inherited or made weak by a way of life. Obviously people have to die of something, and it would be too much to expect all links of the chain to give way at the same time so that life gently and rapidly fades away. Only that could truly be called death from old age.

The disturbing thing is not the existence of the weakest link but that a link is made weakest because it is eroded, and that modern society increases the erosion. It fosters the incidence of degenerative diseases by multiplying the stresses that cause them. Occasional stress can be helpful, for it exercises our adaptive potential. Constant, eroding stress, like a drop of water endlessly falling on a rock, is destructive. It accounts for premature aging and for miserable old age. Old age, even extreme old age, should be active, enjoyable, and healthy. Such is the life of many centenarians in countries where diseases of civilization are not widespread. But this is not so in our world.

Essential Hypertension is not Necessary

Question: What is the most frequent disease in the United States as well as in most advanced countries?

Answer: It is not cancer, nor heart disease, nor arteriosclerosis, nor even mental depression. It is essential hypertension, *essential* meaning, simply, that its cause is not known. Perhaps 20 percent of adult Americans suffer from essential hypertension, and most of them don't know it. This is a frightening figure, one that is substantiated by a number of studies, including one undertaken by the American Medical Association which showed that 4,625 out of a group of 22,929 industrial employees suffered from high blood pressure.

Medically, essential hypertension is described as a disorder of unknown origin, characterized primarily by an elevated diastolic blood pressure, associated with generalized arteriolar vasoconstriction. In plain words, this means that small arteries are being squeezed, so that diastolic blood pressure (that corresponding to the relaxation of the heart muscle) is abnormally high. Systolic pressure, corresponding to the contraction of the heart, also increases.

It is amazing that many people have never heard of or paid attention to essential hypertension and that many doctors don't even routinely check for it. Nobody, after all, dies of moderate hypertension, but countless people die from the diseases hypertension can cause, notably, heart attacks and strokes.

A reading of 120/80 is considered normal for an adult, and occasionally high readings (often at times of stress or after a physical effort) are nothing to worry about, even if you feel your face getting red and hear blood pounding in your head. But a regular elevation in blood pressure, however moderate, exerts a continuous stress, sometimes unnoticed. The effect of hypertension can be compared to the effect of any other form of stress: an occasional stress leads to adaptation, but constant stress leads to erosion. With the continued stress of moderate hypertension, small vessels may rupture, and the overactive heart may become enlarged. The vessels of the kidney may also become damaged. Before long, it is too late. Heart failure, hemorrhage of the retina, kidney disease, or cerebral hemorrhage (stroke) have taken their toll. Essential hypertension may not be easily cured, but it can be prevented, and can be prevented from becoming more severe.

The most important thing for us to remember is that a balance must be struck between too much and too little stress. We must no more become hothouse creatures than harassed nervous wrecks. Unfortunately, industrial civilization seems to be designed to produce both extremes.

Industrial Civilization:
A Dream Become Nightmare

The industrial age exploded with the technical means to adapt our surroundings to our wishes. This was done rapidly, in quick steps taken as soon as technology made them possible and without much consideration of their impact.

No sooner did something become feasible than it was put into practice to modify the environment, to make life easier, to give man the comfort he had been striving for, to give him more, and more, and more things. It was a dream come true that became a nightmare.

It wasn't long before we took for granted what was given us. We complain that the telephone, the washing machine, the car occasionally break down; we no longer marvel that they exist at all. The change was so rapid that some people who are alive today can still remember the time when electricity, gasoline, automobiles, and refrigerators did not exist or were very rare. For some people, these commodities still don't exist.

In man's new home, the cold of winter, the torrid heat of summer, the downpour of rain or hail have vanished to give way to the optimal recommended average temperature and humidity. Today's average apartment has more comforts than the royal palace of 200 years ago. Comfort soon followed man into his automobile and into the subterranean passages he need not leave if he desires to avoid the harsh facts of nature. With electric lights and heat man was even able to replace the sun when it went down and make his days as long as he chose. First radio and now television will entertain him as far into the night as he wishes to give up valuable sleep.

Food is no longer eaten raw and needn't be torn apart with tooth and claws. We shall see later what damage can be done to animals simply by cooking their food. Our food is now prepared, cooked, tenderized, and flavored; preservatives make it easier to keep, colorants give it a pleasing appearance. Thousands of chemicals are also introduced into our food. It is already becoming artificial, and there is talk about making it entirely synthetic.

It has come to be considered quite normal for children to wear braces or to have teeth pulled because they no longer fit their mouths. We know we have gastric problems and that new diseases or syndromes are frequently discovered. We are not quite sure whether these diseases are really new or whether they become known because new diagnostic techniques make it possible to discover them.

In the abundant society, one no longer starves between successful hunts, although one tends to be malnourished. Hunger and occasional fasting were part of mankind's past. Fasting remains as a tradition in nearly every religion, perhaps as a ritualization of something that should not be abandoned, because it is useful.

The fact is that we do not really know what we eat, nor do we know what we should eat. Science has come up with a lot of formulas, but not with the formula of life. We know we must eat proteins, carbohydrates, and fat, but we do not really know all of the elements these contain. Every now and then, some mineral or organic substance is found to be essential to life, and there is usually a press release to announce the discovery. Nevertheless man survived before any of the essential elements were identified. He ate them because they were supplied by nature. Once such an element is identified and synthesized, it can be made available in the form of a pill. But no scientist will claim that we know, or that we will ever know, all of the essential elements that we need.

We do know, however, that these elements, known or unknown, are available in natural food, because if they weren't, they would not have become essential and we would not be here to talk about them.

When we denature natural food, we lose some of these elements. We may be able to replace some, but we cannot be sure we replace *all* that has been lost.

Science has given us a lot, and it shall give even more in the future, but we must recognize that it cannot give us as much as nature has given us. This does not mean we should abandon benefits derived from science, but it does mean we should realize the risk of abandoning nature or going against it.

Food recommended by dietitians may offer the easy, short-term benefits of digestibility, weight loss or gain, muscle building, child-rearing, or whatever other specific purpose may be sought. But its long-term effects are absolutely unknown and by long-term I mean not only the effects on the individual who eats it, but on his children and his children's children.

We cannot give our children better mental or physical inheritance than we possess. But the good seed is not enough. Good earth is necessary.

A child inherits not only from the parental chromosomes that combine when spermatozoon meets ovum. A child's fate is even influenced by the condition of his parents during conception — whether his parents are healthy or sickly makes a difference.

The mother's condition when she carries the child, likewise, can change his destiny. Abuse of tobacco or medicines, addiction to narcotics, or malnutrition have all been proven to cause congenital malformations or fetal death. Our way of life and the food we eat have subtle, and not immediately detectable, influences.

It is true that modern medicine has made possible the conquest of the major plagues of humanity. Vaccines and antibiotics have drastically reduced mortality. The weak are no longer doomed to early death, and the sick can be healed or at least be made to survive to a relatively old age.

All of this sounds fine. The question, however, is whether man is adaptable to the environment he has adapted to his whims?

Striking a Balance Between Stress and Sybaritism

Environment leaves its imprint upon the genetic makeup of human beings, be it through gradual change from generation to generation, or through the selection of the mutations that are best suited to the changing environment.

Now that, for most people in what is known as the civilized world, the struggle for survival is no longer a part of life, we struggle not for survival, but for a better life, or for a life with more comfort and for the possession of more material goods, what is happening to our adaptive potential or vitality?

There is no longer the need to adapt to scorching heat, to high altitudes, to cold, no need to be on the alert for the sound, sight, or smell of an elusive prey, rarely the need for intensive muscular work or endurance. The only requisite for "a good life" today is an ability unknown to our remote ancestors and usually requiring no struggle with a hostile natural environment. It is the ability to *make money*, and it is that very specialized ability, to the exclusion of almost everything else, that controls the selection of the fittest to our new world.

I don't mean there is anything wrong with making money. Money making is a very peculiar pursuit, generally not related to other abilities we have developed during our evolution. If money were clams, you'd have to dive for them. If it were ostrich feathers, you'd have to run for them. But it is nothing of the sort. It is a very simple and, at the same time, a very complicated commodity. You can catch it by sitting behind a desk, or by exercising a very limited number of muscles, those, for instance, needed to dial a telephone number. Of course this doesn't mean you don't exercise your gray cells, but you do it in a very special fashion, one that does not correspond to any evolutionary pattern.

As a result of this, modern man can become something like a peach wrapped in cotton, or a domesticated animal which need not struggle for survival. He has grown bigger, fatter, fulfilled, or at least filled full. But some kind of struggle or effort — physical as well as mental — is indispensable to the formation of a complete man. Look at the beauty, the dignity of a wild duck, and then at the sad picture of a domesticated fowl, overweight and adapted to nothing but the broiler. Domesticated man too has a weak body, and often a weak spirit.

Yet it takes little to reverse this, because within man, dormant perhaps, is the unaltered potential he has inherited from a million generations that have fought for survival. Recognition and avoidance of particular stresses, relief by periodic breaks away from the stressful situation or group, revitalization by the use of simple, usually ridiculously inexpensive natural remedies and foods, discovery of real privacy (unbroken by the marvels of electronics), learning how to sleep and rest, occasional but complete changes of surroundings and occupation are pursuits sufficient to stretch man's vital muscles and slow down the process of premature aging.

I do not advocate total abstinence from stress. Total abstinence from just about anything is excessive, and only greenhouse vegetables lead a completely stressless life. They tend to be tasteless, too. But permanent stress (which is, in the final resort, useless stress), aside from wreaking havoc inside you, leaves no time for joy. Joy is the best of therapies and the best prophylaxis too.

Nor do I advocate abstinence from the commodities made available by modern technology. I would even go as far as recommending the use of electronic gadgetry. Put Beethoven's Ninth Symphony on your stereo (or whatever else represents for you an explosion of joy), forget everything else and let yourself be carried away.

You will have taken a beginning step toward improving your health. There are many more you can take to help yourself.

4. Overweight: A Road to Premature Aging

Overweight is directly related to ill health, loss of vitality, premature aging, and mortality. The statistics on the subject are striking.

The mortality rate among people who are 20 percent overweight is 30 percent greater than that of those who maintain the proper weight. The mortality rate for those who are 40 percent overweight is increased by 70 percent. According to the American Medical Association, one in every five Americans is overweight. When these facts are put together, the importance of the problem becomes evident.

Every person has fat in his body, usually more than he suspects. A trim and well-exercised person may have fat equivalent to 15 to 20 percent of his entire weight. If you are overweight and do not exercise, as much as 30 to 50 percent of your body weight is fat. For instance, if you weigh 175 pounds and should weigh 140 pounds, the 28 pounds of fat (20 percent of 140) you should have and the 35 additional pounds make a total of 63 pounds of fat. Clearly this can mean many people have as much as 50 to 100 pounds of fat, which is too much for anyone.

Fantastic and revolutionary ideas have been introduced to promote weight loss. Some of these, such as an exclusive protein diet, I would hesitate to recommend to my enemies.

According to the Better Business Bureau, the American public is bilked out of several billion dollars every year by fat-reducing quackery. The forms this quackery takes are versatile indeed: reducing pills, reducing belts, reducing machines, reducing diets, reducing creams, reducing injections, and, of course, books to make you reduce through high or low calorie diets, thinking men's or drinking men's diets, high-fat and low-carbohydrate diets, macrobiotic, organic, or grapefruit diets, ad nauseam. Recommending general weight-reducing diets is a hazardous business because people are overweight in different ways and for different reasons. They bear the "overweight" label, but each one is an individual patient with his own problem.

The Four Basic Body Types

Although we have different types of constitutions and individual predispositions toward ill health, it *is* possible to make broad, general classifications of body types to aid in the diagnosis and treatment of weight problems. Granted the classification is simplified, and everybody is a combination of at least two or more types, but even this most superficial breakdown can be helpful. The reader will perhaps recognize in the descriptions that follow the references to ancient astrologic element typing — earth, air, fire, and water — as well as the medieval concept of humours — blood (sanguine), phlegm (phlegmatic), yellow bile (choleric), and black bile (melancholic) — as character determinants. It is no accident that, throughout history, scientists and other observers of the human species have sought to classify and rationalize the various temperamental traits and to make a connection between the mind and the body of man.

There is the ectodermic or asthenic type, symbolized for the ancients by the earth. He is thin, not necessarily tall, often with a prematurely hunched back, with long limbs but not much muscle, who is often shy, reserved, pensive, and brooding, a reader or a student, sometimes with little interest in sensual pleasures. Dominated by his nervous system, he has an active metabolism and often an overactive thyroid. It seems that his favorite season for being sick is spring. He seldom becomes obese. At worst, at some time past his 40's or 50's, he begins to look like he has swallowed a large pea. He is likely to have a bad digestion and occasional ulcers — he worries. Nevertheless, old age will be kind to him, and he will retain much of his vigor and his mental powers. Physicist Robert Oppenheimer was close to personifying this earth man.

Next is the bilious, or muscular type, identified with fire. Athletic, hairy, sometimes swarthy, he is a "supermale," with a firm handshake and a calmness and self-assurance that can bespeak a leader. Women like him. Physiologically, he hyperoxidates, that is, his metabolism is high, he runs on superchargers. Neither shy nor brooding, he thrives in society and likes sports. His weak points are his liver, his kidneys, his digestive system. He must be careful, since in his 40's, there is the risk of a radical slowdown — muscles may turn to fat, he may lose hair, and his cholesterol should be watched. President Gerald Ford and former chancellor Willy Brandt partly fit into this pattern.

The sanguine, or mesodermic type, was associated with air. His muscles, well-proportioned, tend to be covered with a thin layer of fatty tissue, giving him a stocky appearance. He laughs, talks fast, is active and optimistic and usually likes food. His metabolism is rather slow, and his main problems will be associated with hypertension, the lungs, and the heart. Once past his 40's, he should avoid excessive food and drink. The ectodermic type may easily get away with these, but they are dangerous to the mesoderm. He should continue at least moderate exercise and an active professional life, or else old age may be difficult. Winston Churchill was mainly an air person, and so is Golda Meir.

Finally there is the lymphatic, digestive, or round and globular type. According to the ancients, he is water. The legs, often short in proportion to the rest of the body, seem to be designed to carry the bulk of the belly and torso surmounted by a big head. He is an easygoing person, seldom prone to overexertion, but astute. He can be an excellent businessman or politician and feels at home during a meal. He is a slow oxidizer and that's part of his problem of overweight. Everything he eats seems to show, and once it's there, it is exceedingly difficult to get rid of it. His medical problems gravitate around the gastrointestinal tract, and blood circulation is poor. He tends to be sick in the autumn, and the diseases he suffers from may be long-lasting. Hermann Goering, whom I once had the dubious pleasure of meeting, was of the water type. This doesn't mean that water types cannot be perfectly nice and friendly and good-natured.

These are rough sketches, containing many variations and in-betweens, and there are interchanges between one type and another. Yet, they serve as touchstones for the physician in guiding his patient to become his own doctor. For in the treatment of obesity, this is the goal a physician must achieve. He cannot stand behind you every time you reach for the cookie jar or the extra cocktail, and he can only help you reveal your own motivation.

The Mirror Test

If you have a health problem, a good way to start treatment is by having a good look at yourself. I do not mean in your best suit on your way out to dinner or the theater.

Find a tall mirror and strip yourself naked. Resist the temptation to blow up your chest or, if you are a woman, to arch your back or tense your muscles to give a better appearance to your breasts. Start from the top down, and don't hesitate to be cruel. Is your face slightly rounded and puffy, the skin unhealthy-looking? Does your neck remind you of Thanksgiving? Are your shoulders drooping and your back hunched? Is your chest drawn in and flabby, your breasts sagging? Do your muscles no longer possess natural tonus but hang down like draperies? Does your stomach prevent you from seeing your toes without bending over? Fat deposits around the trunk and on the hips and thighs are easy to recognize. If you look fat, it is probable that you are fat and that you need to reduce.

And you go on, below the waist; the rules of the Marquis of Queensberry do not count in this game.

The result of your critical self-examination, most likely, won't be catastrophic. But whether you are 26 or 86, you will perceive some of those telltale signs. You need maintenance, reconditioning, revitalizing, perhaps remodeling. Most likely you must watch your weight or try to lose some. Many factors come into play to make you what you are. Stress, food, ecology, and genetic traits are among the most important. Some of these factors are beyond your control. Our genetic makeup cannot be changed. There is not much that you, as an individual, can do about altering the existing ecology, though there is something you can do about its impact upon you.

Reducing stress, for example, is within your reach. You can either eliminate some of it from your life or learn to cope with it. Food is another major element you can influence. The trick is to know how and to want to do it.

Well-known nutritionist Jean Mayer of Harvard University has suggested that the average American doctor knows slightly more about nutrition than does the average secretary, unless the secretary has a weight problem, in which case she knows more.

This is a severe judgment, but the fact is that diet and nutrition are complex matters, and the medical profession has not yet found the answers to many questions about how the body uses and stores food energy and why different people metabolize at different rates.

Certain facts, however, are known. In order to function, your body needs raw materials — food. From food, it requires carbohydrates, proteins, vitamins, minerals, and fat. Proteins are needed for replacement of tissues, and fats and carbohydrates supply energy. In Chapter 10 we will discuss the role of vitamins and minerals.

The human body can use food in different ways. If you do not eat enough carbohydrates and fat, for example, your body may use protein as a source of energy. This is not the most economical way to obtain energy, but it can be relied on when the quick-energy sources, fats and carbohydrates, are unavailable.

Six Types of Obesity

Each person has his own way of using up, or not using up, food, and therefore there are different origins and forms of obesity. Like the various morphologic types, the causes and types of overweight are seldom clear-cut, but I have observed at least six distinct patterns. There is often an association between two or more of these, but if you are overweight, you will probably find that you are closer to one pattern than to any of the others.

Constitutional obesity

This occurs most frequently with women, and it is the consequence of a specific physiologic change, such as puberty, pregnancy, and menopause. At puberty, young girls frequently pick up a few pounds too many, and some women may experience a transitory weight gain during each menstrual period. Significant weight gains often happen during pregnancy, though this is usually a result of overeating. Pregnant women can be very indulgent with themselves, and so can their husbands. If this is repeated during each pregnancy, obesity can become severe.

But as a rule, constitutional obesity is not a serious problem. It is important for the patient to realize that a moderate diet can help her overcome the problem. Radical, fast-acting diets or certain drug treatments, on the other hand, can aggravate constitutional obesity.

Psychogenic obesity

Psychologic problems can be associated with any form of obesity, but in some people the psychologic aspect becomes predominant. Psychogenic obesity usually originates with a specific stress situation: divorce, death of spouse or close relative, marital infidelity (by either patient or spouse), professional problems, or any other traumatic experience. The number of possible stressors is infinite, but they act in one of two ways: the stress either triggers compulsive and clandestine overeating, or it provokes glandular imbalance.

Sometimes this form of obesity is not readily diagnosed, because the patient hides it. I recall one wealthy woman, in her early 40's, who came to me for treatment. She would have been very attractive if she lost weight, and it seemed obvious to me that her problem was plain overeating. I put her on a very mild diet to begin with and told her maid to be sure to control the amount of food served to her at each meal. After several weeks, there was no weight loss whatever, and I put her on a stricter diet — still without any results.

Then she had an accident. She broke her leg and was forced to stay in bed wearing a cast. She continued on the same diet, but now, though she had no exercise at all, she started losing weight. I was perplexed. Some weeks later, when she could walk again, she started picking up weight. All was explained the night her maid caught her in the kitchen, gulping down some hastily prepared sandwiches. She had been doing this all along, during the entire treatment, except when she was immobilized by the cast.

When I confronted her with this, she burst into tears and confessed that she had emotional problems associated with her divorce. She agreed to try again, but she still did not, or could not, follow any diet.

I then tried to develop a kind of negative reflex in her. I took her to an amusement park and showed her her future in a deforming mirror. I ordered her favorite food, but as she ate it, I tried to associate it with something repulsive. After more than a week of this, I wrote a series of notes with awesome warnings and asked the maid to put one in the refrigerator every evening. It took persistence, but it worked.

When prescribing a regimen, the treating physician should be wary of psychologic consequences. Withdrawing the excessive food is like forcibly taking the thumb out of a baby's mouth or taking away Linus' blanket. Sometimes this can precipitate a depressive condition. In the treatment of psychogenic obesity, the doctor-patient relationship plays an important role, and an attempt to discover the psychologic roots of the problem must go hand in hand with any physical treatment.

Stress can also trigger obesity without a substantial increase in food intake. Little is known about the mechanism of such weight gain except that it involves a disorder of the hypothalamus. Why it is that in some persons stress causes obesity and in others anorexia and weight loss, or ulcers, or headaches, remains a mystery to us.

Professional obesity

I use this term to designate a pattern of overweight which is really an occupational disease. The businessman or salesman who wines and dines associates and customers is a typical example of the professional obese. He is given, sometimes daily and occasionally twice daily, the opportunity to have a gourmet meal, free of charge. He becomes the slightly overweight *bon vivant*, the jolly fat man who, unlike the psychogenic obese, is not a solitary but a social eater, who enjoys every bite as well as the company during the meal. He knows by heart the menus of the best restaurants and is on a first-name basis with the chefs. When he travels, he is likely to select the airline not for the hostesses he'll fly but for the meals and drinks he will be served.

I have seen many professional obese, who carelessly put on weight and often acquire a ruddy complexion around their cheeks and nose, from tiny hemorrhages resulting from abuse of alcohol. As a rule, they come for treatment only when something goes wrong. Treatment is painful for them, because it involves loss of a genuine pleasure. It can also adversely influence their professional lives — what client can enjoy a lavish meal while his host nibbles a lean steak and salad?

Unless this type of obesity is compounded by other health factors, I have found the best treatment is not to eliminate gourmet meals but simply to reduce their size. The loss of weight is gradual and slow, but the regimen soon becomes a habit, and the pleasure of eating remains. I try to discourage before-dinner drinks or at least limit it to one unmixed drink. Plain scotch or a small shot of vodka is less conducive to weight gain than is a dry martini or a manhattan. Best of all is to replace the cocktail with a glass of dry wine during the meal.

Restaurant owners and workers in pastry shops and food stores are other victims of professional obesity, as are night workers (nurses, watchmen) who are not constantly active and tend to nibble to while away the time.

Disease-associated obesity

The following are among the major diseases associated — sometimes as a cause, sometimes as a result, sometimes both — with obesity: diabetes, hypertension, kidney disease, gout, menstrual difficulties, gastrointestinal disorders, and cardiovascular diseases. Obesity radically increases the mortality risk of some of these conditions. There are also sometimes contradictory factors: constitutional obesities, for instance, are frequently associated with low blood pressure, but in other cases of obesity, there is high blood pressure, and loss of weight can lower it.

Many diabetics are subject to obesity, apparently as a result of insufficient metabolism of sugars. Once the chain reaction is triggered, obesity compounds diabetes and diabetes compounds obesity. A well-balanced carbohydrate-restrictive diet can give spectacular results in both conditions.

Respiratory problems are compounded by obesity. The weight of the abdomen reduces the use of the diaphragm for breathing, breath becomes short, and lung volume gradually shrinks. Here, too, treating the obesity can greatly improve the respiratory deficiencies.

Glandular obesity

Obesity resulting from glandular imbalance is the *only* sort that should be treated with hormones, and then only when there is no other way of reestablishing hormonal equilibrium. Cushing's syndrome is a typical example of glandular obesity. It results from oversecretion of adrenal glands, and obesity is localized chiefly around the hips and neck. Hypertension is an associated phenomenon, as are skin problems and sometimes excessive virilization. Cushing's syndrome is very difficult to treat, since it is caused by an excess, not a shortage, of a hormone. Myxedema, on the other hand, results from glandular shortage. It is not a true obesity and responds to thyroid treatment. In young boys, obesity can be associated with genital underdevelopment.

One of the most difficult types of obesity to treat is wherein fat deposits characteristic of one's sex occur in isolated areas. For instance, all women tend to gain weight around the hips, men around the stomach or the neck. When the gain of weight is limited exclusively to these areas, diet does not help. It reduces weight all over the body, and the localized excesses become even more apparent. In some cases, exercises can be helpful.

False obesity

The false obese is typically an actor, politician, or other public personality, one whose appearance seems (or is) of paramount importance, and who as a result has become a compulsive weight-watcher. As the name implies, the false obese is not really obese and may not even be overweight, but he thinks he is or is prone to be and so starts developing a sort of nutritional frigidity or impotence, depriving himself of the legitimate joy of a good meal.

The false obese is easy to recognize: he is usually narcissistic, carefully dressed and elegant. He is careful to present himself in his most advantageous position. I remember an actress who had a particularly beautiful profile. For four or five consecutive visits, she managed to find an excuse (strong light, uncomfortable position, and so on) to show me only her profile, except for brief glimpses of her full face. Through habit, she had even developed a very charming sideways glance that could be maintained throughout a long conversation. I warned her that she might end up not only with real weight problems but with eye problems too.

Not only do the false obese deprive themselves of natural healthy pleasures, but they prepare the grounds for very real, and almost instant, obesity. After years of self-imposed rationing, their organism learns to take advantage of every morsel it is granted, and relaxation of the regimen (resulting from a traumatic experience, stress, or simply from giving it all up) precipitates a spectacular, and sometimes fatal, weight increase. This risk is incurred by professional models, who must maintain an unnaturally low weight, and who can indulge in acrobatic fluctuations as the fashion swings from the stringbean to the full-bosom look. (Fashion designers are responsible for much misery and sometimes ill health. They are, unfortunately, out of the realm of the Food and Drug Administration.)

I remember one such patient very well. She was in the garment business when I met her, but she had once been a professional model. Even though she no longer needed to be slim, she still had drastic eating habits. Then one day, an advertising agency asked her if (for a goodly sum) she would model some bathing suits, and she agreed to come out of retirement for this one assignment. The pictures were taken and she was paid, but the photographs were never published. The advertiser found she was too skinny and that her bones stuck out unpleasantly.

She couldn't believe it, until I went over the photographs with her and pointed out angles on her body that she could not see. She immediately decided to gain weight, and I prescribed a very mild weight-gaining diet, to make sure she wouldn't gain too much too fast and end up with a problem of obesity. The following year, she tried again (perhaps to reassure herself), and if you read fashion magazines, you have probably seen her perfect figure displayed in some brief but colorful bikinis.

The Overweight Child

Obesity in children can have severe consequences, and parents should realize that children, too, can and should be put on diets if they are overweight.

Many studies carried out in several countries show that overweight children almost always become overweight adults. It seems that when children become overweight, there is an increase not only in the *size* of fat cells but also in the *number* of fat cells, which is not the case when adults become overweight. Once the children grow up, it is much more difficult for them to lose weight than for people who become overweight after having reached maturity.

A child's diet, however, is serious business. His nutritional needs are greater than an adult's, as he must keep growing. A physician should *always* be consulted before putting a child on a diet, for malnutrition is a real danger.

Overweight and "The Pill"

In recent years it has been observed that women who take birth-control pills are occasionally prone to sudden weight gain. Even if a woman has taken the pill regularly for one or two years without having any weight problems, it can arise unexpectedly. The mode of action of the pill is complex and not completely understood, but there is no doubt that it can trigger obesity, just as it can trigger hypertension. This is confirmed by the fact that cessation of use of the pill, sometimes even without a diet or with a very mild one, is often followed by rapid weight loss.

5. On Preventing Obesity, Low Blood Sugar, and Using Diet Drugs

When an overweight person decides to lose weight, he assumes a responsibility that is, in the final analysis, his own. He must be sure that he knows the causes of his obesity, he must be careful about the methods he chooses to lose weight, and he must have the self-discipline to change his eating habits, at least to some extent.

To prevent, eliminate, or at least curb the problem of overweight is an essential part of revitalization therapy, because overweight represents precisely the kind of stress that is damaging: continuous, relentless taxing of our adaptive potential.

There are almost always emotional problems — either as a cause, or as a consequence — related to obesity. Remember that your doctor is not only a medical expert but also a man you should be able to confide in. This will help you, and it will also help him find his way through a maze that can be very complex indeed. If you find him reluctant to listen to you, consider consulting another doctor. Don't forget that if a mistake is made, you are the victim. But don't abandon professional medical help, which is always better than turning to a crazy fad.

Mistakes in this area are so easily made. I have made many myself and probably will make more. But it is much more pleasing for a doctor's ego to correct other doctors' mistakes than to have his own corrected. The following, classical example will serve to indicate the sort of mistakes often made in prescribing a reducing regimen and will also give you an idea about my approach to the individual and his weight problem.

A patient of mine was an active, dynamic salesman who, in his 40's, suddenly started to gain weight. At first he wasn't much concerned. He did try to eat a bit less and to continue exercising. He played golf and occasional tennis, and still he continued to gain weight. In a few months, he had picked up five or six more pounds, and so he went to see his doctor.

The doctor told him that a radical diet for a few weeks might solve the problem. He gave the man a calorie chart and told him to cut down on starchy food and to reduce his total calorie intake to 1,200 a day.

The salesman was determined and stuck to the regimen and, within days, started losing weight. He had been warned that he wouldn't have as much energy and that he might become tired easily. He observed this to be true.

A month and a half later, having lost about 10 pounds, the man's weight no longer changed. He hadn't quite returned to his normal activity, but his doctor told him to gradually add carbohydrates to his diet to refuel his energy. He did this, and although his daily caloric intake remained well below average, he rapidly started gaining weight again.

When I met him, he had regained nearly all of the 10 pounds he had lost. He was a man of medium size, stocky, dark-haired, and rather short-limbed, but not disproportionately so. Well-spoken and self-assured, he fell almost exactly into the "bilious, hypermuscular type," who often hyperoxidizes. Hyperoxidation is an indication of a rapid metabolic rate. (I noticed he had rather large ears. I have observed that people with large ears tend to prefer bulky food and vegetables, while people with small ears favor more concentrated food and meat. There's nothing scientific about this, and I have no explanation to offer. I just happened to notice this and ever since have found it to be confirmed in about 75 percent of cases, which is, as statisticians put it, "significant.")

After talking to him, the picture became clear. He regularly ate a great amount of cooked vegetables, which have little caloric value but significant volume. During his intensive dieting, his metabolic rate quickly adapted, dropping down by 20 or 30 percent. This is not unusual. During World War II, many physicians in Europe observed that food shortage could reduce basal metabolism by as much as 50 and even 60 percent.

With a slowed-down metabolism and reduced exercise, he nevertheless first started losing weight, but much of the weight loss was muscle and not fat. (This is, unfortunately, a frequent phenomenon. An easy way to determine whether a person has too much fat or just a great deal of muscle is to drop him into a swimming pool. Muscles sink, fat floats. A more scientific way is to use calipers for the measurement of skin folds.)

The addition of carbohydrates, which was not immediately followed by the return of his normally high metabolic rate, produced a rapid weight gain. And the gain consisted of fatty tissue, not muscle. He was back to where he started, but now even more of the overweight pounds were fat instead of muscle.

This is the typically disastrous result of a regimen based exclusively on limiting caloric intake. The result can be even worse when this is accompanied by medication, such as thyroid extract or anorexic pills to reduce appetite.

For such a patient, reading health menus and following standardized regimens can be of little help. A regular, monotonous diet deprives the organism of the ceaseless variations that put to work its adaptive energy. Changes and contrast can liven up the organism's task and give it a chance to adapt variously and to avoid the risk of maladaptation in a single direction, of which this man had been the victim.

The type of person, the reasons for his overweight — glandular, mental, genetic, nutritional — his nutritional habits and preferences make it impossible to recommend a single weight-reducing diet for all. The fact that many doctors and the myriad of diet books propounding fad diets do prescribe diets which fail to recognize the essential differences in people's weight problems is one of the great tragedies of modern medicine. Once again, treatment of the whole man has been ignored in favor of the simplified and, alas, more lucrative across-the-board prescription of whatever diet is currently in vogue.

The Crenelated Diet

In attempting to solve this man's problem, I followed the crenelated or stepladder method I often use that can be varied to suit each case.

Grapes were in season, and I first put him on a brief, three-day grape cure. This means eating little else but grapes. They provide enough energy but require the body to draw on fat reserves. They also help eliminate some toxins. With the grape cure, my patient lost very little weight, less than two pounds.

Then, the idea was to achieve gradual loss of weight in steps which not only would let his organism adapt to the change but also would convert some fat-weight into muscle-weight.

He began with four or five days of rapid-reducing diet, of which there are many varieties. In this case, I prescribed for three days only the egg-and-tomato diet, in which an unlimited amount of eggs and of tomatoes can be taken, in six daily meals. Added to this was a quart of water every day, to help eliminate more toxins. This produced a weight loss of four pounds.

I next put him on a regimen which would cause him to gradually regain some weight, though not all of the four pounds. I told him to eat as much as he wanted of certain types of food:

beef, lamb, veal (with all visible fat trimmed), lean fish (baked or broiled), all types of seafood, chicken and turkey from which the skin had been removed, eggs, cottage cheese, pot cheese, and farmer cheese, and tea or coffee with artificial sweetener. Only during lunch, and in limited amounts, he was allowed starchy food such as potatoes, but could have green vegetables and salads as much as he liked.

This second diet, which was not too severe, continued a balance of proteins and sugars, as well as small amounts of fatty material, and gave him sufficient energy to resume physical exercise. Of course he did gain weight but most of this new weight gain was muscle, not fat.

Five or six days later, when he had regained three out of the four pounds he had lost during the short but fast-reducing diet, he returned to it again, losing four more pounds in two days. Then, I switched him again to the richer diet with its gradual gain in weight and muscular buildup. But every time, between weight gain and loss, there was the loss of about a pound. Thus, within a few months and without feeling like a weakened martyr, the man lost the 10 pounds he needed to lose, but lost them gradually, without upsetting his metabolism.

This crenelated or stepladder type of regimen is even more desirable when the required weight loss is thirty pounds or over. Not only is a rapid diet traumatic, but the results are often ungainly, leaving behind flabby curtains of unfilled flesh.

But diet is not all. We have seen that emotions alone can trigger a sudden gain of weight. Emotions also play an important role in loss of weight. We should never forget the mind-body unit and the feedback between its two component parts that sometimes leads to catastrophic snowball effects. Obesity is only one link-syndrome in the chain of reactions, but it is a very important one in the abundant society that is ours. It is frequently the first step in the degenerative process of premature aging.

It is a confirmed fact that moderate dietary restrictions (and occasional fasts), as well as the consumption of live, natural foods, are healthful and contribute to prolonging the lifespan.

No sensible person denies this, no more than we deny that smoking increases the incidence of lung cancer. Yet I — and perhaps you — smoke. We do it knowingly and accept the risk.

But I find it difficult to accept that we impose risks *we* may be willing to take on persons who are not aware of them and who cannot make a choice.

I mean children. It is bad enough that children in large cities are provided with an annual dose of a few hundred pounds of dust and smoke and assorted poisonous particles in the air they breathe. We may not, as individuals, succeed in reducing this sort of pollution without a long-range and concerted effort. But you and I, as individuals, can prevent our children from being exposed to harmful habits, most significantly those having to do with nutrition.

Prevention of Obesity in Children

A tendency toward obesity is not always easy to detect in children. Some heavyweights simply possess a stocky structure. Temporary weight gains, between the ages of 18 and 24 months, for instance, are not important. They tend to disappear when the child walks and becomes more active. But persistent obesity in children is dangerous. Obese children are the fathers of obese adults.

The most difficult to treat are genetically inherited obesities. A child can become obese without overeating, or else he cannot help overeating, given a chance. In such cases, it is likely that one or both of his parents have a tendency to obesity. Even if neither parent is obese, the combination of genes inherited by the child can predispose him toward obesity. The genetics of obesity are not as simple as those of diseases such as mongolism or straightforward enzymatic deficiencies. Not only can obesity be provoked by an association of different characters, but each of the characters contributing to it may depend on a great number of genes. The earlier such a predisposition is detected and treated, the more easily the consequences are avoided.

Whether the children are predisposed to obesity or not, encouraging children to overeat is one of the most dangerous but common errors made by parents. Modern mothers seem to have retained the ancestral fear of undernourishing their children. A well-fed, which often means overfed, child is considered a healthy child. This is all the more unfortunate since we now know the profound effect childhood eating habits can have on the adult. The tendency to a large appetite, the cravings for sweets and/or carbohydrates are almost always preferences developed in childhood. These preferences are difficult for the adult to modify. Perhaps more important, we know that the number of fat cells produced during childhood tends to remain constant thereafter. A fat child will have great difficulty dieting to become a slender adult.

Let us not forget that evolution has enabled us to cope with shortage, not with overabundance. This applies to children as well as adults. Too much food often produces not a strong child but a "butterball" or "fatso" to his innocently cruel school friends. Such added humiliation can precipitate catastrophic psychologic reactions.

Remember your child will grow, and his health problems will grow along with him. Give him at least a chance to try some untreated, live, natural food, rather than letting him yield to television advertising which promotes additives (to which some food is occasionally added) in order to reach for the premium coupon at the bottom of the box.

I suggest a small experiment, the results of which are devastating. Next time your child loses one of his baby teeth, put it in a glass filled with a carbonated soft drink. Within a few days the tooth will have been eaten away. Microorganisms that cause dental cavities work only in the presence of sugar elements, such as those contained in this drink which is consumed by the truckload by Americans, adult and child alike.

The Role of Sugar

Whatever the reasons for overweight and eating disorders — be they clearly emotional, clearly physiologic, or an unfortunate combination of the two — the overweight American suffers also from a particular excess in his daily diet which in many cases amounts to an addiction. I am speaking of refined sugar. This chemically treated, denaturized substance finds its way, in enormous quantities, into nearly all prepared foods and is added to many others by sweet-toothed Americans. It adds thousands of unwarranted calories to the daily diet and taxes the adaptive mechanisms of the body.

There is an incredible, wonderful constancy in the chemical composition of body fluids, particularly of the blood. This *milieu intérieur*, as physiologist Claude Bernard has called it, is the primeval sea which we have taken along in our arteries and veins. Each change in the *milieu* means a message is transmitted from organ to organ, gland to gland, giving the necessary instructions so that the constancy is maintained.

The *milieu intérieur* is wonderfully adaptive, but there are limits. One limit is being violated with such persistence and to such a degree that something must finally give in: the normal tolerance for sucrose. In addition to natural sugar supplies found in fruit and vegetables, people in some industrial countries consume as much as one hundred pounds of refined sugar per person per year. This means about a third of a pound of sugar a day.

Our organism is equipped to maintain in the blood a certain level of sugar. The antisugar artillery is found in the pancreas, in the form of islets of Langerhans. When there is an excess of sugar in the blood, these cells produce additional insulin, a substance which allows the cells to take up sugar and turn it into energy. When these cells are not sufficiently active, the result is diabetes, basically a dangerously high blood-sugar level which must be fought off with injections of insulin to burn it away.

But the Langerhans cells can also become overactive. So enormous is the constant introduction of pure sugar into the organism that these cells can become overresponsive. In goes the sugar — in cakes, sweetened coffee, sweet drinks, whatever else — and out of the pancreas comes insulin to destroy the invader. The overactive pancreas becomes so well trained to secrete insulin that it starts oversecreting it regularly. The enemy is vanquished but the result is another one: excessive insulin.

Then until the next massive sugar invasion, the body fluids are deprived of it but saturated with insulin. The result is the same as occurs when a diabetic overdoses himself. This is a serious matter because excessive insulin can produce shock and collapse and, on a lesser level, general nervousness, irritability, and anxiety. Doctors have become aware that many mental diseases are simply the result of excess insulin and low blood sugar, both resulting from too much sugar in the diet.

It is amazing that this problem has only recently been recognized with all of its implications. A major study, written for laymen, of low blood sugar (hypoglycemia) and its dangers was published in the United States in 1969 by a nutritionist, Carlton Fredericks, and a physician, Herman Goodman. Yet, in spite of overwhelming evidence, sugar consumption habits in the United States haven't changed much. We have witnessed, instead, the suppression of the use of cyclamates in food and beverages, suppression based on far less conclusive evidence than that existing against sugar (some of the cyclamate research was financed by the sugar industry). A wiser legislation, from the viewpoint of health, would have been to ban not cyclamates but some of those overprocessed drinks too rich in *refined*, denatured sugar.

Low blood sugar has become so widespread that a six-hour glucose test, in my opinion, should be performed routinely and periodically on people in most industrial countries. And a balanced no-sugar or low-sugar and low-carbohydrate diet should be prescribed to a huge number of people as a preventive measure aginst the damage with which they are threatened.

Low blood sugar, however contradictory it may seem, is treated with a diet reducing the intake of sugar and carbohydrates, which are rapidly transformed into sugar. The idea is to give just enough sugar, in frequent, small doses, to maintain a blood level, without the high intake that overstimulates the Langerhans cells. This may mean six or even eight meals a day for a while, but it is well worth it to bring the whole system back into order.

It seems clear that low blood sugar is much more dangerous, and much more common than had been recognized. On the other hand, there has been a temptation in recent years to attribute fatigue, weakness, and dizzy spells to low blood sugar, without confirming the diagnosis by a glucose test and eventually by other hormonal assays and tests. This also can be dangerous, particularly if adrenal cortical extracts are used for treatment.

Diets and Drugs

Before ending our discussion of obesity, I should like to comment on the use of drugs to aid weight reduction. You will have noticed that the dietary approach I have recommended makes no use whatever of appetite depressants, diuretics, or the like. I believe that modification of eating habits, good exercise, and an attempt to understand the root causes of overweight and poor eating habits are the keys to attaining ideal weight. Under no circumstances should reducing drugs be self-prescribed. In those few instances in which a doctor feels a pharmaceutical aid is needed, I would recommend that more than one opinion on the matter be solicited.

With this warning in mind, let me briefly outline some reducing aids which are currently in use.

Diuretics

These preparations are made to help you "pass the waters." For long-term weight loss, they are completely useless, as they can act only on the weight elasticity of the overweight person, that is, the margin within which he can tolerate dehydration. Diuretics can cause the loss of four or five pounds of *water* — and nothing more. As soon as you stop taking them, you will regain this water-weight.

An unpleasant side effect of diuretic treatment (as well as salt-free treatment) is an excessive secretion of aldosterone, the hormone that helps you retain sodium and eliminate potassium. This can result in electrolyte imbalance, a very serious condition.

A mild, brief diuretic treatment can be useful to clean up the organism of some toxins. This is best achieved with a natural method, such as the drinking of cherry stem infusion for two or three weeks are described in Chapters 9 and 10.

There are exceptions, and all of them can only be determined by your physician after a careful study. Diuretics may have to be used, for instance, when obesity is compounded by salt and water retention, usually resulting from cardiac or vascular insufficiency. Otherwise, even if diuretics do no physiologic damage, they only serve as a crutch. For a few days, it looks like magic, but no magic can cure obesity.

Anorectic drugs

Like diuretics, these appetite-reducing drugs are a crutch, and I would use them only in exceptional cases with patients who have extremely limited will power. Not only can these drugs be addictive; they also have frequent undesirable side effects: insomnia, hyperexcitability, vertigo, a prolonged feeling of dryness in the mouth. They eliminate the need to face the causes and problems that underline obesity and do nothing to alter eating habits or prevent the return of a weight problem.

Thyroid hormones

They are occasionally prescribed in the treatment of obesity, but they should be used only if it is clearly demonstrated that obesity is associated with thyroid deficiency. Once thyroid hormone has been used unnecessarily, obesity seems to become particularly resistant to more conventional treatments.

I could list a few other drugs, but their fashion is usually short-lived. Dinitrophenol, for instance, was once boosted as a potent weight reducer, and indeed it was. It acted on the cellular level, interfering with oxidation and formation of ATP, the energy-transporting molecules. Unfortunately it was so potent that it was also toxic, and its use resulted in a number of deaths. Scopolamine aminoxide was advertised as a weight reducer, because it produces drowsiness and thus helps a person to refrain from eating too much. It was withdrawn from the market, but other chemicals that produce drowsiness are still used as ingredients in weight-reducing drugs. Benzocaine, a local anesthetic, was included in another drug, on the grounds that the anesthetic effect on the stomach and intestines would reduce appetite. This drug, too, has been withdrawn following a court order.

There is good reason to be suspicious of *any* drug advertised as an effective treatment of obesity. The problem of obesity is so widespread, the solution so difficult, that a really effective drug, one that would not be dangerous at the same time, would not require a single inch of advertising to become a worldwide best-seller. You would find out about it not from advertising spreads but from scientific journals and front-page headlines.

Obesity is an aging factor. The maintenance of your ideal weight through a natural and varied diet and reasonable exercise is a building block to revitalization. There are no real secrets of good health, no magic formula diets. Rather, the key lies in understanding the psychologic and physiologic bases of the problem and establishing a regimen which takes these individual specifics into account.

6. Sex: A Key to Vitality and Longevity

The association between sexual functions and longevity is well-established.

Sex is a normal function, like eating and breathing. One of the differences between it and other vital functions is that you can survive without sex, whereas you cannot survive without food or air. Nonetheless, a sexless life shortens the life span. It deprives the organism of the powerful peaks in hormonal secretions that accompany sex, and it deprives man and woman of one of the most fundamental, most natural, and healthiest joys that exist.

Sex is also a particularly fragile function. This is understandable from an evolutionary viewpoint: if anything goes wrong with an organism, it is better for the future of the species to avoid passing on the defect to future generations. However, as man has evolved and civilization has advanced, sex has become more than just a reproductive function aimed at the survival of the species.

Some primitive societies have never made the association between sexual intercourse and childbirth. The nine-month lag between one event and the other is a long one, filled with many other events and ceremonies that could be considered causative of childbirth. When one of our primitive ancestors grunted his equivalent of "Eureka!" and tried to explain that if you put this into that, nine months later you have a child, he may have been regarded with the same skepticism as was Einstein when he first talked of relativity. His people might have argued that sometimes you put this into that and you get nothing, and sometimes you do it and one month later you have a child.

Sex and reproductive capacities are powerful tools with which to manipulate men. Witch doctors, priests, and other leaders of primitive societies quickly assimilated sex into religious ceremonies and created taboos and regulations, generally making the whole business less spontaneous and more complicated.

Our Judeo-Christian cultures have long considered sex for purposes other than procreation to be a sin. For complex reasons that belong in a theologic treatise rather than in a book on medicine, sex came to be the most heavily penalized of all human pursuits. Good food, music, admiration of works of art are sensorial activities accessible even to monks, but sex became the snake of sin, and the rearing of its ugly head, even in thought, opened the door to purgatory, at the very least.

In the last few decades, the situation has changed again. This is not, however, the first sexual revolution mankind has witnessed. In the past, as in the present, the results have been rather favorable. In ancient Greece, there were periodic sex cures. (I have used the term "cure" in connection with such therapeutic regimens as the grape cure or juice cure, and it is one that I prefer to "orgy" or "bacchanalia," which have naughty implications.) It was also a time when mankind produced some of its most beautiful works of architecture, sculpture, painting, and literature and developed a profoundly human type of society, a truly participatory democracy of a sort that is difficult to achieve in our more complex world and in our huge cities.

Sex and a Ripe Old Age

Even on the individual level, an active participation in sexual endeavors has long been credited for prolonging and enhancing human life. Myths and legends abound of fruitful oldsters. It is no coincidence that these people were as well known for the large families they produced as for the length of their lives.

One of these record-holders is Old Thomas Parr, an Englishman who, according to legend, was born in 1483 and whose tombstone in Westminster Abbey indicates 1635 as the date of his death. Old Parr is probably a hoax. Many suspect that Thomas Parr had a grandson of the same name, although the famous surgeon, William Harvey, who was the first to describe the circulation of the blood, upheld the age of 152 after an autopsy.

There is an intriguing aspect to Parr's story. After performing the autopsy, Harvey noticed that Parr had particularly well-developed and heavy testicles. The no-less-famous Swiss revitalization therapist, Paul Niehans, always argued that longevity was related to the secretion of the endocrine glands, notably the sexual glands. He believed Parr's longevity was due to his heavy testicles and prolonged gonadal secretion.

There is some logic to associating longevity and reproductive function. Nature, as a rule, is more concerned with a species than it is with an individual, and in this respect, man's role on earth is finished when he has exercised his reproductive faculties and raised his young. It is not illogical, then, to suspect a link between reproductive sexual activity and the overall life span. Once the propagation of the species has been assured by the required number of impregnations and births, the animal should presumably make room for the next generation.

A striking example of this is the Pacific salmon. It swims often for thousands of miles across an ocean to deposit its eggs in some predetermined spawning grounds. When doing this, it is a powerful machine, colorful and with a smooth and brilliant texture, strong enough to swim upriver in spite of rapids and waterfalls. But once its last mission has been accomplished, it ages within two or three weeks. It loses teeth and muscle, the skin becomes rugged and patchy, the flesh seems to draw tighter around the bones. The fish looks and acts old.

There is no doubt that the relationship exists and that continued sexual function, both in men and in women, is one of the contributing factors to vigorous old age. I wouldn't go as far as an Argentinian colleague who maintained that men are not impotent because they are old, but that they grow old because they are impotent. This doctor has designed an ingenious prosthesis to assist failing erection (and asks $8,000 for the equipment). But premature interruption of sexual activity and of the secretions of the sexual glands does accelerate the aging process in both men and women.

Some Early Practitioners of Sexual Rejuvenation

In the last few generations, our Western world has also acknowledged the association between sex and healthy longevity. Cell therapy, practiced today as a clinical revitalization technique, is discussed in Chapter 20. However, it is interesting to note that some of its early experimental applications were, as is true today, in the area of sex.

In 1889, Charles-Edouard Brown-Sequard, professor of physiology at the University of Paris, made an announcement to the French *Société de Biologie*, which can be considered a milestone in the annals of revitalization theory. A prestigious personage even at age 72, Brown-Sequard occupied the chair formerly held by the great physiologist Claude Bernard.

Brown-Sequard first announced that he believed weakness in old men was caused in part by the decrease in the function of their sexual glands and gave himself as an example: "I am 72 years old. My natural vigor has declined considerably in the last 10 years."

After whetting the appetite of his audience, he came up with a *plat de résistance* that the aging members of the *Societé de Biologie* (average age above 70) could not readily digest. Brown-Sequard told them he had ground up the testicles of young dogs and guinea pigs, mixed them in a saline solution, and made an extract of the juices. After some preliminary experiments, he started injecting the stuff into himself.

"I have rejuvenated myself by 30 years, and today I was able to 'pay a visit' to my young wife," he concluded. There was considerable uproar. The press publicized the discovery, and, in order to answer the sudden demand, Brown-Sequard set up a nonprofit organization to prepare and distribute large amounts of bull's testicle extract.

Brown-Sequard was on the threshold of discovering hormonal therapy, but his extraction methods were not sufficiently developed to obtain significant amounts of male hormones. The scientific community turned thumbs down, his wife left him, and Brown-Sequard, who might have been remembered as a pioneer in endocrinology, left Paris in disgrace and died shortly thereafter.

The idea was picked up in 1890 by Eugen Steinach, an Austrian physician who theorized that if he could stop the testicles from producing spermatozoa, the crucial hormone-producing part of the testicles would be more activated. To do this, he tied off the vas deferens, the sperm ducts, believing that the spermatozoa would back up and stimulate a greater hormonal secretion. This theory was never verified, but his operation, now known as vasectomy, became a fad (and is still with us as a male contraceptive technique) until another new star rose.

Dr. Serge Voronoff was a dynamic, cultured, multilingual Russian aristocrat who had practiced at the court of the Egyptian Khedive. The well-supplied harem there was guarded by the traditional eunuchs. Dr. Voronoff found that these castrated men were a rather sickly lot who aged more rapidly than other men and never lived long. This is well known, and it is one of the arguments favoring the relationship between an active sex life and longevity: castrates (and this includes psychologic as well as surgical castrates) have never held longevity records. It can be noted, incidentally, that eunuchs, although many of them were learned and cultured people, have never become great leaders, artists, or creators. A goodly supply of hormones seems to be a prerequisite for these achievements.

Voronoff concluded that if the deprivation of sexual glands could accelerate aging, an increase in their production would have the opposite effect. Returning to Europe, he developed a technique, which later became world famous in organ graft and transplant surgery. He extracted the testicles from young animals, sliced them into small pieces, and then implanted the slices under the scrotum of an older animal, attaching them next to the capillary supply of the testicles. Transplants made between animals of the same species would take, and Voronoff obtained some excellent results, which he announced at the 28th French Surgical Congress in Paris in 1919. Voronoff unhesitatingly used the word "rejuvenation." Participants in the congress were invited to have a look at some animals, old rams and a bull, he had rejuvenated.

The public reaction was much the same as had been accorded Brown-Sequard when he announced his injection treatment. Voronoff's work was potentially more interesting, because if a transplanted bit of organ could take, the treatment would act not as a one-shot hormone injection but as a permanently increased source of hormones.

Voronoff started treating human patients. He rightly thought that the use of young human testicles would give the best results, but religious and legal considerations made it impossible for him to obtain testicles from young men who had died accidentally, and he turned to man's closest relative, the chimpanzee.

He set up a clinic in Italy, near the French border, and in the 1920's more than 1,000 elderly men visited him to receive implants of slices of chimpanzee's testicles.

Voronoff's idea was not without logic, although we know now that there was no chance for the transplants from one species to another to take permanently, because such foreign tissue is rejected in what we now refer to as the host-versus-graft reaction. Between the two living tissues the reaction was strong enough to reject the implant. At best, there may have been a transitory effect similar to that of a hormone injection, as the bits of testicle contained active hormones, but no permanent rejuvenating effect could be obtained. One of the major drawbacks of Voronoff's technique was that transplants from chimpanzees with subclinical syphilis could infect the patients.

Voronoff's work was criticized by the scientific community, but it stimulated hormone research and undoubtedly contributed to the eventual treatment of sexual disorders with hormone injections.

Use and Abuse of Hormones to Increase Sexual Potency and Treat Menopausal Symptoms

Such injections are frequently used today. Sometimes they are warranted, too often they are abused. They have two main shortcomings: they create a dependency, and they also create lazy endocrine glands. Glandular secretions work on the feedback system. Shortage of a hormone in the blood is registered by the anterior part of the pituitary gland and the hypothalamus, which in turn secrete other hormones in minute quantities. When these hormones, circulating in the blood, reach the gland to which they bear the message, this gland follows the orders and starts secreting the missing hormone. When the hormonal level in the blood rises, the anterior pituitary and the hypothalamus send a message to stop production. Artificial introduction of a hormone overtakes this cycle, and the gland that is supposed to do the work no longer needs to. There are sufficient hormones in the body and no need for the pituitary to give any order at all.

In the 1930's, natural testosterone was isolated, and later, it was synthesized. Testosterone injections not only renew lagging sexual capabilities in patients who really have a deficit of the hormone but also encourage the buildup of tissue and cellular reproduction.

By that time, even skeptical gerontologists had to agree that there was a rejuvenating effect — or, better perhaps, a revitalizing one. Testosterone injection for men is really the only universally accepted therapy to extend youth, but it is not widely used because of the shortcomings mentioned earlier and because there is an underlying fear (never really confirmed) that testosterone injections may increase the incidence of cancer.

Nonetheless, hormone therapy as regards sexual potency is in its infancy, and as we shall see later, there are infinitely better, natural ways to achieve the same results.

Women experience a problem that is quite different from that of men, not only because their hormones are different (estrogens) but because women are radically and suddenly deprived of these hormones during menopause, as the ovaries become atrophied and stop producing them. Aging is more sudden. A side effect of this is increased susceptibility of postmenopausal women to arteriosclerosis (hardening of blood vessels). Estrogens have a protecting effect against arteriosclerosis that has been demonstrated even in men. In severe cases, the risk of breast development in a male patient is preferable to the risk of heart failure.

Estrogens are often used for the treatment of menopause-related disorders in women. The results are about as good, and the shortcomings about the same, as in the use of testosterone injections for men. Again, there are better ways, particularly if one becomes aware of them early enough. Fortunately, we are living at a time when such therapy encounters a favorable climate.

Sex is for Health

The point is not to avoid hormone therapy but to postpone it for as long as possible by exercising vigorously the function that is closely related to these hormones. This function, clearly, is sex.

During sexual activity, increased amounts of sexual hormones are secreted. They circulate in every part of the body. If male and female hormones could be dyed with chlorophyll green, we would all appear to be Martians, dark green in spots, lighter in others, but green all over to the tips of our toes. And growing darker green during sexual arousal.

This is the best hormone injection you can have — your own.

Let us start by wiping away some cobwebs.

Sex is no sin. It is good for you, unless it is bad for you. Anything related to sex, anything that makes it enjoyable, is good for you, unless it does harm to anybody, whether yourself or your partner.

So, there is sex for pleasure, and it also turns out to be sex for health.

How ridiculous are some traditional sayings, such as that sex exhausts you, that orgasm empties you of life forces, that excessive sex will debilitate you, that masturbation will make a drooling idiot of you. It is comparable to saying that using a muscle will waste it. Of course sex will tire you, just as prolonged muscular activity tires you, but it also trains you and your glands to perform better and more often. An active sex life is one of the best youth preservers. Frequent sex is absolutely harmless. The worst that can happen if you habitually make love through the night is that you will be sleepy in the mornings. And this problem can be solved by shifting some of your sexual activities to daytime.

It is wonderful when two people are in love and stay in love. It is a state of grace, and in this state, sex is a particularly rewarding experience. But not everybody is fortunate enough to be in love all the time he is capable of having sexual relations. I see no reason why two people who are not in love, but who are attracted to each other or simply feel they would like to have sex together for the pleasure of it, shouldn't have it. When they do, it is not unlikely that they *will* start loving each other. The introduction of feeling is almost inevitable in sexual relations, and it enhances them. This is why, perhaps, we speak of "making love."

I believe that the real meaning of the so-called sexual revolution is these: that people can meet and make love for pleasure, without having to feel guilty about it and without having to hide it as something sinful or antisocial; that it is quite normal for people (married or not) to explore all the possibilities of sexual pleasure, without limiting themselves to the once prevalent attitude that "sex-is-for-reproduction-only."

This revolution has been particularly kind to women. For too long, woman has been held up as the passive object of man's performance, and it was generally denied that she is as entitled to pleasure as is man. Many women have never had an orgasm in their lives, and there was a time they could do nothing about it. Now they can.

This is a wonderful thing, for women as well as for men. Men have limited orgasmic capacities, but the time has come when women can take advantage of this fact instead of being the victims of it. Until some time ago, a woman who admitted to multiple orgasms was considered to be either hysterical or a nymphomaniac. In fact, the nymphomaniac is quite the opposite: she goes on and on in her obsessive pursuit because she cannot have a truly satisfying orgasm.

Sexual excitement curves

Man and woman have entirely different sexual excitement curves.

Man's rises sharply and quickly to reach a heightened and pleasurable plateau, the preorgasmic peak of his excitement. This pleasurable state can be continued for a very short — or a very long — time. Men who are too quick don't enjoy the full spectrum of the sexual experience. They feel the approach of "the point of no return," a point on the plateau just prior to orgasm when nothing can be done to stop it. The solution is to delay reaching the point of no return as long as possible. With training and the cooperation of one's partner, this can be learned fairly easily, because when one senses this point approaching, there is still time to delay it by stopping for a few seconds, or changing rhythm, or by concentrating on giving pleasure to your partner while holding off your own. It is amazing how many people have never really tried to prolong this plateau! I am not a sex educator, but I have found myself, more than once, in the position of teaching an intelligent 60-year-old man to become, for the first time in his life, a good lover.

For a man, this plateau of excitement ends with orgasm. The curve drops sharply and rapidly back to its lowest, pre-excitement point. It can start rising again after a recovery period, the length of which varies with the individual and the circumstances.

In woman, the picture is entirely different, and the very understanding of this difference can transform a couple's unexciting sex routine into a constantly rewarding adventure.

Woman's curve starts rising gradually and slowly. It takes her, as a rule, much more time to reach the peak of her excitement. By then, her partner has most likely already reached his. If he's an inexperienced lover or a cad or (very exceptionally) really incapable of holding his peak long enough, he'll have an orgasm before the woman has reached the peak of her excitement and is ready for one herself. If this pattern is repeated frequently, a woman may be rendered frigid, or she may seek satisfaction elsewhere.

Once a woman reaches her peak of excitement, she may soon be ready for orgasm. But, unlike man, her orgasm is not followed by a sharp drop. She is soon ready for another. If a man stays on his peak long enough, she will have had several orgasms by the time he has his. When intercourse ceases, the woman is still high on her excitement curve, and while the man, who has dropped to the bottom of his, turns around to reach for a cigarette, she still vibrates. This deserves consideration.

The erogenous zones

Lovemaking should not completely exclude any senses. Just as every part of your body is alive with sexual hormones, so every part of your body, not just your genitals, participates in lovemaking.

We know a few precise erogenous zones: the breasts (both male and female), the back of the ear, the inner part of the thigh. But the entire skin is erogenous. And though a man requires at least some genital stimulation to achieve orgasm, a woman can have a complete orgasm without her genital organs being as much as touched.

And let us not forget the body-mind relationship and unity,

which is crucial in sex. An enormous part of sex (when it is something higher than the satisfaction of the simple need to empty one's testicles) is not only receiving but giving pleasure. It is a perfect illustration of the feedback principle, so universal in biology. This leads to very exciting possibilities and discoveries.

7. Solving Sexual Problems and Dysfunctions

Impotence is one of the most frequent complaints of men who come to see me for treatment or advice, or who have been clients at revitalization centers, such as Renaissance. For women, the complaint of frigidity is somewhat less frequent. Many women accept frigidity as an immutable fact, and by the time they have matured and aged, they have so completely given up that they don't even think about it. Men also, in their 60's and 70's, sometimes accept sexual inadequacy as a normal result of aging; there is an unfortunate social context encouraging this.

Naturally there are differences between the sexual performances of a 20-year-old and a 60-year-old man or woman. But strange as it may seem, not all of the differences are to the

disadvantage of the older person. It is well to see these differences in their proper light, so as not to consider them the telltale
signs of sexual decrepitude.

An older man does not perform as frequently. In fact, the
highest quantity-performance potential is at puberty. Two or
three years later, the frequency of sexual performance has already started to decline.

However, there are reasons to believe that an older man's sex
life is as, if not more, satisfying to himself and his partner.
Erection is slower, as if more thoughtful. The tightening up of
the scrotal sac is not as pronounced, and pre-ejaculatory lubrication (from glands other than the testicles) is not as active. But
once the older man has reached the peak of sexual excitement,
as pleasurable as it has been at any age, he can bask in it at
length, without worrying about going, unexpectedly, beyond
the point of no return and thus to rapid ejaculation. Even without training in the arts of sex, the older man's experiences have
given him much better control. In a duet, where both partners
are active, he easily harmonizes with his partner. When he takes
the pleasure-giving role of solo performer, he has excellent mastery in bringing the greatest joy out of his partner as instrument.

In many cases, the point of no return disappears. From the
extended peak of his plateau, the man goes into the final
ejaculatory stage. The volume of seminal fluid is reduced. The
prolonged peak, aside from being pleasurable, has the revitalizing effect of sending male hormones pulsing through the body
and of keeping the glands exercised.

The recovery period, however, is longer than in younger
men. He will not be able to have a second erection as rapidly as
he did as a young man. Rather than considering this a debility,
the older man can take advantage of his capacity to retain peak
excitement for a long time. This can be the opportunity for trying some variations. In a duet performance, he can easily provide his partner with several orgasms.

Orgasm and ejaculation aren't the only purposes and pleasures of a man's sex life. Too often a woman feels inadequate if
she hasn't led her man to ejaculation, and a man, by feedback,
feels inadequate for not having achieved it, even if he has
thoroughly enjoyed the rest of it.

Some readers may think it coarse for me to speak of sex in old age with such seemingly clinical detachment. But the subject is usually overlooked, and ignorance, combined with the unfounded belief in the inevitable decline (and fall) of sexual powers, has done too much harm as it is and has deprived too many people of the joy and the benefits of a harmonious sex life. One's right to a healthy and full sex life should be claimed along with one's right to a healthy and full life; it is part of it.

I should like to tell a story that I think is beautiful and that represents a satisfying experience in the life of a physician concerned with *total* revitalization.

It happened at Renaissance not long ago. A couple came for a 10-day revitalization course. He was a successful businessman in his 60's, and his wife was about 10 years younger.

There was no mention, at first, of sex problems. They were tired, harassed, needed to get away. They could both benefit from embryotherapy, cell therapy, and additional tonifying treatments (thalassotherapy, skin treatment, relaxation training — all of which we discuss in later chapters).

At first I met with both of them, but as soon as the treatment started, the consultations became individual. I learned that they had been married for well over 20 years and had three married daughters.

They were married when the wife was 27. She had had an extremely strict religious education, and when they met, she was still a virgin. He had been married three times before. They fell in love, flirted, petted, and some of these petting experiences brought her to orgasm. She remained a virgin until they were married but hadn't mentioned this fact to him. He never asked but assumed she had had some previous sexual experiences. Romantically, she reserved her virginity as a kind of wedding gift.

On the day of the wedding, he had a few drinks too many. When they retired after the social festivities, he expected her to be a sexy volcano, and, after minimal conversation and minimal foreplay, he took her violently. The experience was painful to her. On the previous occasions, she had felt high excitement with him and even orgasm, but this first marital experience left her cold, injured, and profoundly disappointed.

He promptly realized this and gently tried to erase the wall that had come between them. She refused varied sexual foreplay, because she had been taught that it was dirty and evil. She came to consider sex as strictly for reproduction and soon forgot the glimpses of pleasure she had known.

She had three children who had to be cared for and brought up, business problems had to be dealt with, and the couple went through more than 20 years loving each other but having no full sexual relationship. During all that time, she hadn't had a single orgasm. He had a few extramarital experiences that had not been very successful. He loved his wife.

When I met them, both had completely given up. I spoke with her privately first.

"It's no longer a problem," she said. "I don't even have to put up with it any longer, since he has become impotent. Everything is settled."

"Would you mind it," I asked her, "if you regained the ability to enjoy sex, to be able to have a normal orgasm?"

"I would. I don't want to," she said. It seemed to me she was relieved that the whole matter was over and that she could simply dismiss the problem.

She next told me something that surprised me. Now that the children were married, she had decided to get a divorce, either to live alone, or perhaps to remake her life with a man better suited to her.

When I talked to him, his case appeared to be clearcut: it was secondary impotence, first specifically directed at his wife and then generalized to other women.

He didn't "turn her on," and consequently, she no longer turned him on. He had been married before and had known satisfactory mutual sex relationships. His wife, he said, was sexually inactive and considered his demands as an ordeal. He, too, confided that he was considering divorce.

"Did you really try to educate her?" I asked him.

He said he had, but that his approaches had been rejected as "dirty." I saw them alternately during the medical treatment, and I asked her if, after all, she wasn't sorry to be throwing away the love they had for each other and suggested it might be worth trying to make another go at it, including the renewal of a harmonious sex life.

"What good is it? At his age, he has become impotent."

I told her that the treatment he was following might do a lot of good and that she might try teasing him a bit. She was shocked.

Two hours after that consultation, she asked to see me. She just wanted to tell me that, perhaps, I was right, but that she hadn't the slightest idea of how to go about it.

When I saw him, I made the same suggestion. "What's the good of it?" he objected. "I have tried so often."

On the following day I saw them both together while they were having lunch. I suggested they shouldn't leave Nassau without driving to the west end of the island to admire one of the island's magnificent sunsets.

"And when the sun sets, why don't you hold hands?" They blushed. They said something about not having held hands for years. In midafternoon I saw him alone in my office. I warned him that he should not, under any circumstances, make an aggressive pass at her nor suggest intercourse. He said he couldn't anyway. A few weeks earlier, in desperation, he had hired the services of a prostitute to see whether he could at least have erection. He couldn't.

They drove off to see the sunset. Shyly, he took her hand, feeling like a schoolboy on his first date. The sunset, I was told, had been exceptionally beautiful. After a while she put her hand around his neck and teased his ear.

On the following day, he told me he had felt paralyzed and lost; this simple contact had brought about a complete erection. But he didn't dare make a move toward her, fearing that it might break the spell or that she would withdraw.

I wasn't quite sure by then whether I was Hippocrates or Cupid, but I recalled that she had complained of some rheumatic pain and, changing subjects, told him that unfortunately the nurse was off at night and that perhaps he could soothe her with an aromatic ointment I had prepared.

Later, when I saw her, I told her the same story and mentioned that her husband should replace the nurse at night. She said it would embarrass her. "Turn out the lights," I said.

We were coming to the end of the ten-day treatment — there were only one or two days left. For the following night's massage, I described some erogenous zones on her body and suggested that he rub them with gentleness but some insistence.

The next day she came and told me that the massages had been very pleasant. "You could, perhaps," she ventured, "prescribe some ointment I should use on John?"

I did and asked her whether he had had any erections. "How in the world would I know? You don't imagine I *look* there, or that I touch him?"

I said that a small gesture would be enough to find out. She didn't answer but mentioned that they had decided to stay on a few extra days after the treatment was officially over, just as a vacation.

They stayed for three weeks altogether. I saw them occasionally, but thought it unnecessary to have further clinical conversations with them. So we spoke of rain and shine. A wink he gave me once was sufficiently explicit, and so was the glow around his beautiful wife, who looked ten years younger. And I do not ascribe this to the medical treatment. Facing the problem, being away from day-to-day worries and routine, a sunset, and perhaps a bit of innocent medical trickery had given this couple the full, enjoyable, loving sex life they had been deprived of for some *20 years*. The problem had been solved; the only pity is that it hadn't been solved earlier.

Is this, you may wonder, such a typical case? Are sexual problems really solved so easily? In fact, most are. Not easily sometimes, sometimes without a tropical sunset, but always with a lot of understanding.

Solving Sexual Problems Yourself

What are, in fact, the major sexual problems? The serious study of sexual problems is only recent. Much has been done by William Masters and Virginia Johnson of the Reproductive Biology Research Foundation in Saint Louis, Missouri, authors of

Human Sexual Response and *Human Sexual Inadequacy*. Masters and Johnson admit they have dealt with only a fraction of the problem, but at least they have begun the inquiry, and they have made significant advances. They have given us facts, which have sometimes been criticized, not with the help of other facts, but with unproven ideas. Unfortunately, the Masters and Johnson books and publications are not very readable for the layman (or even for the physician) but they have tremendous reference value. (Fred Belliveau and Lin Richter have "translated" Masters and Johnson's works for the layman in their book *Understanding Human Sexual Inadequacy*.) Most important, in the experience of Masters and Johnson, 82 percent of human sexual inadequacies can be cured.

Unfortunately one doesn't always know where to go to have these problems treated. The Reproductive Biology Research Foundation isn't around the corner for everybody, and sex therapy clinics are still rare. Your doctor, unless he has taken a particular interest in this, may not be of great help. This is an area, however, where you can help yourself but it requires some knowledge of the matter, a mind unencumbered by prejudice, and, usually, a cooperative partner.

The first thing to realize is the location of most sexual problems. It is not below the belt but above the neck.

Of course, there may be some physiologic causes to the problem. For women, a defect in physical structure, such as a very resistant hymen or a relaxed vagina, are medical problems which can usually be resolved with minor surgery. Diseases such as infections and tumors are treated medically, and the lack of adequate lubrication can be overcome by the use of a lubricant, such as Vaseline. This lack is often the result of psychologic rather than physiologic reasons, and the use of the lubricant need not be permanent. Sexual function, once normalized, helps trigger natural lubrication.

Frigidity

The only real problem for a woman is frigidity, resulting from mental blocks. This condition is widespread, but statistics have little significance, since many women do not admit frigidity though they live with it through their married and sexually active (or, in this case, passive) life.

Girls who have been raised with the idea that there's something sinful, evil, or improper about enjoying sex, who have been told that sex is to have children or "to make your husband happy," often develop a resistance to orgasm. Even after they have consciously overcome the mental attitude at the origin of frigidity, the subconscious block persists.

The last thing to do about frigidity is to accept it as an established fact you have to live with. Whether you have what is called "primary frigidity" — that is, you've never experienced an orgasm in your life — or "secondary frigidity" — you have, but at some point you've stopped — chances are you can break away from it. Psychiatry or analysis can help, but such treatment can last for months or years, and there are easier ways, unless a psychiatrist succeeds in determining rapidly the origin of your frigidity. In some cases, knowing the origin may be enough to eliminate the problem. The reason passes from your subconscious to your consciousness, where you can deal with it more easily.

Secondary frigidity may be caused by an incident that might seem unimportant. You may have had one single unhappy sexual experience: a rough and painful defloration; sexual relations with a man you dislike but yielded to because of liquor, mood, or a group situation; a homosexual experience you feel guilty about; or an unwanted pregnancy or an abortion. There are thousands of possibilities — it would be impossible to list them all.

Primary frigidity usually goes back to childhood, although in some cases it has been provoked by the first sexual encounter.

Frigidity caused by hormonal imbalance is extremely rare. Even dwarfs can enjoy sex, and even after menopause, when the ovaries stop functioning, the libido is not affected. Libido in women, in fact, seems to be dependent on male hormones — women have some male hormones, just as men have some female hormones. The major risk after menopause is shrinkage or loss of vaginal lubrication from lack of intercourse.

I should discuss, perhaps, another form of frigidity: compulsive passive (as opposed to active) lesbianism. There is no moral judgment involved in this opinion, although sexual perversion is usually described as behavior not enjoyed by the writer himself, and this is behavior I have obviously not enjoyed.

All people are somewhat sexually ambivalent, not only from the endocrinologic viewpoint but because they can respond sexually to stimulation by people of either sex. But exclusive passive lesbianism — when a woman cannot respond sexually, not to mention reach orgasm, with a man — is definitely a form of frigidity. Very often it is also the *result* of frigidity, particularly secondary frigidity provoked by a rough, brutal man who has "turned off" the woman to other men and caused her to seek sexual satisfaction with the gentler sex.

Such exclusive passive lesbianism can be cured if the woman wants it. If she does, a gentle and patient approach on the part of her male partner will be most helpful.

Active lesbianism is another matter. Most active, male-role lesbians don't want to become heterosexual, and not wanting it is the obstacle that puts an end to treatment before treatment can even start. For instance, experiments have shown that men who wanted heterosexual activities, but had failed in their attempts and could engage in sexual activities only with other men, could "learn" to be heterosexual. (This is true also of fetishism, when sexual activity is focused on an article of clothing or part of the body.) The treatment consists of instructing the man to masturbate (using whatever fantasies he wishes for arousal) and then, just at the moment of orgasm, to switch his fantasy to a scene of himself with a woman, or to look at a photograph of a woman, during the orgasm itself. Once he can do this, he is instructed to conjure up the scene a little earlier, and earlier again next time. After a while, the reward of the orgasm, accompanied by the heterosexual intercourse fantasy, brings him to the point where the heterosexual fantasy or image can arouse him. Then, gradually, heterosexual intercourse can be introduced.

Even if you cannot discover the origin of frigidity, it doesn't mean you cannot cure it. Many women who cannot reach orgasm during intercourse can achieve it by masturbation, but there is no reason for them to limit themselves to this satisfaction and be deprived of sexual enjoyment with a partner.

The best way to treat frigidity is, of course, to do it with the help of a man you love. First, the understanding should be sufficient for you to be able to talk to him about it frankly. If he does love you, he will try to help. Clinical treatment can also be successful with a surrogate partner. In any case, an empathy must exist, or develop, between the partners.

The man's role is of paramount importance. He should realize that he holds the key, and he must use it with infinite care.

If you are still shy, you can start on your own by exploring your body's potential. Do not try to immediately reach a climax through masturbation but try to find which stimulus most excites and pleases you. Don't think about useless, and sometimes false, notions like the respective values of clitoral and vaginal orgasm (a meaningless Freudian invention), but try to recognize your most pleasurable pattern. Don't be afraid of it.

Then introduce it into lovemaking with your partner. The man, above all, should be gentle and patient and careful not to trigger a negative reaction. He should become sensitized to a woman's slightest vibration or stiffening because it may be the only clue that something's wrong. Young girls are warned by their parents that "petting starts where it stopped last time," and this is the pattern to follow in this gradual thawing. Attempting to go too fast may bring you several steps backward, losing terrain you had gradually gained.

Finding the solution to frigidity is a man's work, and one cannot overemphasize that patience is the required virtue. It is much better if the woman become eager and impatient because the man is too patient. It's worth waiting for. Once you break through the barrier, the cure is good for life. (The same gradual approach is necessary for a woman to train for multiple orgasms. Once she has learned, she will become a lifelong adept or addict, but the addiction is not dangerous.)

For women, as for men, prolonged sexual abstention should be avoided, particularly after middle age. Masturbation, or the use of a vibrator, can be useful to avoid too lengthy disuse. The use of lubricants, available in jelly form, can prompt the return of natural lubrication.

Vaginismus

Another female sexual problem — fortunately rare but potentially very unpleasant — is vaginismus, the involuntary spastic contraction of the vaginal outlet, where the muscles tighten and close. Sometimes it is so severe that penetration cannot be made. Or if the spasm occurs during intercourse, the penis is caught in the trap, swollen with the blood that made the erection possible. The effect can be compared to the replacing of a champagne cork — except that it hurts.

In many cases, vaginismus only occurs when the woman receives a shock of some sort during intercourse, such as fear or surprise. In others, it can be a more permanent disorder, occurring every time the woman attempts intercourse, so that, for instance, a marriage cannot be consummated. In the latter cases it becomes, in effect, female impotence: she cannot be penetrated.

Vaginismus is not a physiologic disorder. Like frigidity, it is typically psychogenic. Sometimes it can be associated with extremely severe religious taboos on sex inculcated during childhood, with a psychosexual trauma, or with painful intercourse. However, psychotherapy is not always effective in the treatment of vaginismus. The Masters and Johnson clinic uses dilators of assorted sizes that are progressively introduced into the vagina, sometimes to be kept there for several hours at night. In their experience, this treatment has never failed.

On the whole, sexual inadequacy in woman is represented, in a vast majority of cases, by frigidity. And it is also, in a vast majority of cases, completely and much more easily curable than is generally believed.

The most unfortunate and, alas, widespread attitude is to regard frigidity as a permanent, irreversible state — the failure of orgasm is regarded in the same light as the loss of a tooth or of an organ. This has been the greatest obstacle to successful treatment. Women give up and often hide this curable inadequacy behind a simulated orgasm for fear of appearing inadequate or of being rejected by their partners.

Thus knowledge of the near-certainty of a cure is important, not only to the woman but also to her man. There is hardly a man who would not be willing to control himself and show some patience, if he knew he could help change the sexual life of his woman from the dreary play-acting she has imposed upon herself to a full, enjoyable, natural sex life — with a feedback reward coming to him.

Loss of libido

There is, of course, one requisite to a healthy, joyful, rewarding sex life, and it is the same for women and for men: libido — the desire to do it, the interest in the opposite sex.

Loss of libido usually results from a general loss of vitality, from stress, from disease, or from unhappy sexual experiences. Libido *does not* naturally disappear with age, and when it disappears (whatever the age) it can be regained.

Usually libido persists longer than capacity, but sometimes loss of libido triggers loss of capacity. This can happen in young and old: the death of a spouse, a disappointment, or even an overwhelming interest in something else. Then disuse leads to dysfunction, and dysfunction reflects itself upon the general state of health.

Loss of libido seems to be less frequent in man than in woman. But in man, sexual inadequacy seems to be more frequent than in woman, and it takes a greater variety of forms.

Why is it so?

I think that at least part of the answer is that man is expected to perform. A woman, if worse comes to worst, can "close her eyes and think of England." A man can't. Patriotism won't make the flag go up, and when it doesn't, the inadequacy has additional feedback because the woman obviously is aware of it. Even if she's nice about it, it doesn't subtract the insult from the man's injury.

Premature ejaculation

Ejaculatio praecox (premature ejaculation) is one of the more frequent forms of male inadequacy. It occurs regardless of age. The ejaculation comes quickly, unexpectedly, and not so pleasurably — in most cases before penetration.

A classical cause of this is the initiation of a young man by prostitutes. Prostitutes as a rule don't want to lose time, which means more customers to them, so the faster the better. Hurried along in this momentous experience, the young man is flustered, and a few rapid manipulations can produce ejaculation. This can become a chain reaction: eagerness to penetrate, and anxiety not to, create a premature reflex.

Deliberate, controlled masturbation, far from being harmful, can help overcome this, particularly if it is performed by a sympathetic partner who understands the problem. Or the woman, aware of the problem, can play solo, trying to dominate the reactions of her instrument, man. She should not drive toward ejaculation, but only try to keep erection as long as possible. With enough empathy and experience, she can tell orgasm is approaching and stop at that point. If she cannot sense this point, an indication from her partner will help. This is particularly effective on a second erection, when there is, as a rule, less of a rush.

Once ejaculation has been controlled, you try to enter, if only to reassure yourself you can. But at this stage do not strive toward ejaculation — withdraw and enter again. Your visits can become more frequent and longer. Gradually increase the number of strokes, still trying to avoid ejaculation. With a patient partner (and patience doesn't mean she is willing to remain unsatisfied and frustrated — there are several ways of taking care of that), the problem can usually be overcome.

Masters and Johnson have developed a more radical method which they have found to be successful in cases of premature ejaculations: the squeeze technique. Squeezing the tip of the penis immediately stops the urge to ejaculate. The woman can do this by placing her first and second fingers on the superior part of the penis, near the tip, on either side of the coronal ridge, and the thumb on the inferior surface, opposite the two fingers. Rather strong pressure must be applied for three to four seconds. The ejaculatory urge disappears. Shortly afterwards, the woman can start stimulating it again (sometimes the erection will be slightly diminished after the squeeze).

The man himself can apply the squeeze or direct the woman to do it when he feels the ejaculation is imminent, and he can press her fingers to show the pressure that can be used without being painful.

Ejaculatory incompetence

The opposite form of sexual inadequacy, also associated with psychologic causes, is ejaculatory imcompetence. The difference is that the man usually maintains his erection and has no problem in penetrating the vagina, but then he cannot ejaculate— — although he can *after* withdrawing. This is in most cases associated with the subconscious denial of his seed. Sometimes it happens with a single partner (often his wife) while intercourse with others may be normal. Obviously this is associated with mental trauma of an origin as varied as can be most forms of impotence: fear of causing pregnancy, severe religious objection against the use of contraceptives, or, generally, association of ejaculation with some unwanted or feared event.

This can be easily treated. Men suffering from ejaculatory incompetence can usually ejaculate when masturbating, and the easiest approach is for the woman to perform this, gradually learning the sensitive points, and eventually completing the masturbation when the penis is partially inserted.

In my experience, I have never encountered a case of either premature ejaculation or ejaculatory incompetence which could not be treated. But if they are not treated, they can lead to true impotence — the inability to achieve a serviceable erection.

Impotence

Misunderstanding, anxiety, shame, feelings of inferiority pile up to make any form of impotence increasingly hopeless. Impotence, like VD, has a connotation of hidden, shameful disease, and this contributes to the deterioration of mental and physical health in countless men.

The irritating thing about it is that it is curable in nearly all of the cases, unless there is an underlying physical cause, which is rare. The quicker you act, the more rapidly you will get rid of it.

There is a simple test to determine if impotence is curable: if, at any time, during sleep, when excited by erotic pictures or literature, when waking with a desire to urinate, when kissing or petting a woman, you can have an erection, your impotence is curable. Whether you are 50, 60, 70, or older, if you suddenly find you are impotent, don't give in to the belief that it is the end of the line — unless, of course, there is an underlying disease, in which case you should consult a doctor. In some cases, obesity, diabetes, or some anticoagulant drugs can have this effect, but then, most likely, you wouldn't have an erection at any time.

Like frigidity, impotence can be either primary or secondary, and the causes are of a similar nature, except that for a man, there is an added one: fear of poor performance. Unfortunately, this is encouraged by some of the current pornographic fare, which leads you to believe that if you can't perform every time with full success and if you don't do it with the efficacy of a stud horse, you're not quite a man. I would rather hold the opposite view: someone who has 100 percent efficacy isn't a man — he's closer to the stud. Although some may consider this to be a compliment, I don't.

Excessive religious orthodoxy, traumatic experiences during childhood, incestuous connotations in relation to one's mother, disappointment in an affective relationship, guilt feeling are among the principal causes of primary impotence.

Impotence is considered secondary when the man had performed adequately but later became incapable of doing so. Among the many possible causes, fear of performance again predominates. Excessive excitement can cause transitory non-performance: the first opportunity with a much-desired woman or the wedding night are typical examples. This is not impotence but a mere incident, and a normal one at that. It should not be overemphasized (by either partner) lest there be a feedback reaction that really turns it into impotence.

Women should be particularly understanding and cautious about this. I insist on this point, because a woman's attitude can provoke an impotence that could so easily be avoided, just as a man can provoke frigidity. Men, even more than women, can suffer from the negative feedback because it is so evident to *both* partners when something goes wrong. As I have said, women can get away with it, but men can't. In men, with occasional exceptions resulting from fatigue or excessive consumption of alcohol or tobacco (tobacco is a powerful antiaphrodisiac), fear of failure to perform is the cause of a majority of cases of impotence.

The best way to treat impotence is to eliminate the fear of

nonperformance by demonstrating that performance is possible. This may sound like a contradiction, but it isn't.

I have found that the most effective way of doing this is by telling the patient — and, if possible, his partner — to go through everything that is associated with sexual activity but to stop before completing intercourse. During treatment you must come to accept the fact that intercourse and ejaculation are not the purposes of the loveplay you are about to engage in. Everything you are about to do will be pleasant, and you can do anything you feel like that isn't harmful to you or your partner, except engage in intercourse. If there is an erection, let it stay up or go down, admire it or encourage it, but no more.

The purpose of this is more than just to give you confidence in the fact that you can have an erection. When an erection is carried to its plateau and maintained there without ejaculation, it prompts an increase in hormonal secretions. As I have said before, these hormones are far better than an injection; they flex your hormonal glands, while an injection makes them lazy. I have found that the best and most definitive results are achieved when this is repeated, keeping the erection as long as possible, without letting yourself go as far as ejaculation. After a few days, the hormonal buildup is fantastic.

In this treatment, the woman takes over and learns to control the man's responsiveness. He becomes the instrument. She can, at this stage, use a very effective trick: gripping his sexual organ with hers. To do this, she must learn to control the principal muscle of the vagina, the pubococcygeal muscle. This can be learned by trying to contract it voluntarily. If it doesn't come naturally, she can learn it in the bathroom, while urinating, by trying to interrupt urination several times. Once it is learned, this control becomes a strong additive to both partner's pleasure during intercourse.

When the man has succeeded in maintaining a good erection several times, intercourse is permitted. I prefer to give the green light myself, but reasonable, patient, and loving partners can do it on their own just as effectively after having decided not to take advantage of the first opportunities to have an ejaculation.

Obviously, a man can't cure impotence on his own nor with a

prostitute, and it is difficult with a new conquest. The treatment must be carried out by two people; a woman you take home for the first time might be taken aback by the request if you have the courage to formulate it, and the prostitute is generally incapable of or unwilling to feel any empathy.

Masters and Johnson have found a novel solution to impotence that shocked some people when it was first heard about. They employ surrogates — women therapists who volunteer to play the role of wives or lovers. This has been quite effective and has become an accepted way of treating impotence when neither a wife nor a willing partner are available.

Another way to treat impotence that is still in the experimental stages is biofeedback. Some men can learn to will an erection, something that cannot normally be done and that usually has the opposite effect when attempted without prior biofeedback training. We shall discuss biofeedback in Chapter 16, but basically it is a technique for mastering some so-called involuntary functions, such as brain waves, heart rate, and blood pressure, and it can apply to erection. Expert yogas can will an erection just as they can slow down their heart rates, but I find that the possibility is rather unattractive. Reaching an erection via normal excitement and foreplay would seem more satisfactory, but this is a personal opinion. As Saint-Exupéry might have put it, if you are thirsty, one of the pleasures is to walk slowly toward the well and to listen to the wheel sing as you draw the water.

In my opinion and experience, the most satisfying sex life is one shared by two people completely open to each other. There is no friendlier thing people can do together than make love. It is also a private part of life from which outside interference, taboos, social standards, and laws are excluded. Statistics should be excluded too: do not compare your performance to that of others (whether real or presumed), not even with the Kinsey Report. Do it your way, at your rhythm and your frequency, but if you like it, do it, and do not stop, whatever your age.

8. Learning to be Good to Yourself: Your Spirit, Emotions, Intuition, and Mental Outlook

Books about health speak of diets, blood formulas, heart conditions, kidney stones, drugs, and other subjects of medical and scientific research and practice. They seldom speak of the spirit, an entity largely ignored by modern science. The spirit cannot be isolated, quantified, or synthesized. Science has made attempts to penetrate its secrets, and is making more every day, with the upsurge of interest in ESP and other unexplained "powers" of the mind. However, though the spirit, or soul, or inner self (or whatever you wish to call it) is beyond the grasp of scientific analysis, it is a most important part of the human equation.

We share with the rest of the animal kingdom the possession

of hearts, legs, livers, and brains. Some animals have heavier brains that possess more nerve cells than those of human beings. They seem capable of emotions, and sometimes display what appears to be nobility of character, devotion, and selflessness. But it is evident there is a difference between man and animal in this regard. This question — of the existence or nonexistence of the spirit — has been the subject of countless dissertations, which I do not intend to review. Let us accept the scientifically unproven postulate that the essential prerogative of man over the rest of the living world is the possession of a spirit.

In my opinion, the single most important aging (or youth) factor is in the mind. It may be impossible to measure the mind or spirit, but it is not difficult to illustrate its strong influence on other systems and organs in the body. Moral, intellectual, and emotional activities are linked with the highly complex nervous and glandular systems as well as with other organic functions. A slight modification of glandular secretions or the injection of additional hormones can profoundly modify the mental state of a person. The mental state, in turn, can profoundly modify glandular secretions and the general state of the organism.

The Powerful Emotions

Emotions act on organs and glands. One pales with anger, flushes with pleasure, turns green (yellow would be more accurate) with envy. Strong emotions can alter completely the state of the organism, more often from health to disease than the opposite. Emotions alter the blood formula, nervous equilibrium, digestion, circulation, and hormonal secretions. The measurement of the changes in glandular secretions, and to some extent even of the organism's electric currents, can even gauge the intensity of an emotion.

During any type of stress, as Dr. Selye showed, the endocrine system naturally secretes large amounts of ACTH; ACTH may facilitate our adaptation to stress, or it may help us get away from it. This emotion-generated excess of hormones can have a direct positive or negative effect on the body. The relationship is not completely understood, but its existence is beyond any doubt. Experiments have shown that when ACTH is injected into people, they develop a sense of well-being and euphoria, then excitement and insomnia, then depression. A striking example of this was given in an experiment conducted by the CIBA Foundation. Given ACTH, a pianist with limited technique could suddenly start playing, with unexpected brio, difficult works that had been inaccessible to him before. As the effect wore off, he progressively relapsed into mediocrity again, and then into depression.

Hormones, in effect, are self-made drugs, yet we are seldom warned that through our mental activities we can overproduce certain of them and bring repeated unfavorable action to ourselves. Obviously if we seek the euphoria, and want to avoid the depression, unwittingly we will seek out stress, to ensure there will be no opportunity for the third, natural, letdown stage to take place. We will veer constantly between the euphoria and the insomniac stages, using up our valuable — and limited — stress adaptive potential much too quickly. Stress is simply not a natural state. During stress, sex glands shrink, and a woman's monthly cycle becomes irregular. Gastric and duodenal ulcers occur much more frequently in people ill-adapted to their work or way of life, and who suffer from tension and frustration.

On the other hand, we are not told that our mental activities can also bring the errant production of hormones back into order, and produce a favorable action to our organism. We can do this by creating a favorable emotional environment, actively pursuing the positive for ourselves, and finding joy.

Trusting Your Own Intuition and Judgment

Almost all of us have, on our own, knowledge and intuition that should not be rejected because it is not measured or because it does not yield statistically significant or scientifically substantiated results.

Intuition, the judgmental mechanism of the spirit, has been given us to use and to develop. Genius, including scientific genius, uses all means at its disposal. Without intuition to illuminate the path to deductive thought, scientists such as Galileo, Newton, Einstein would not, each in his time, have revolutionized science.

Also, we should not reject empiricism, the teachings of our own experience. Medical dictionaries tend to identify empiricism with quackery, forgetting that medicine is always empiric, as well as scientific. When a doctor prescribes aspirin against a headache, he does so because in his experience and that of others, it has been found that aspirin can relieve a headache. Not because he can give a scientific explanation of how aspirin works.

We know instinctively that certain emotions are good, others are bad, that certain things are ugly, others are beautiful. We can usually tell the difference between the positive that is good for us, and the negative that is harmful. Knowing what hurts has, in itself, therapeutic value. It has even more value when this knowledge is consciously put to use.

In life, we sometimes feel propelled in a certain direction, following a pattern imposed by society, and we follow this path with as much inertia as a satellite launched into a predetermined orbit. Generally we pursue fame, money, status, success, with disregard for the ethical, moral, or emotional harm we may be doing to ourselves or others. We do not always do what we know or feel to be right or good because it does not seem as important as these other values. What we do not realize is that it is vitally important.

After all, "humanity" is a trait of the human species, and the trait is not new. In his book, *Choisir d'être Humain*, biologist/philosopher René Dubos observed that tenderness and altruism have deep roots in our biologic past. He noted that the first complete skeleton found of a Neanderthal man, who lived some 50,000 years ago, was that of a 60-year-old arthritic, so deformed that he must have been incapable of hunting or taking part in other activities. If he survived to such an advanced age, although useless to his clan, it must be because he was cared for, perhaps tenderly, by others. Other similar examples are known from archaeological findings.

It is perfectly normal to act rightly not from altruism but from egotism. Egotism is inherent to life, be it on a cellular, individual, racial, tribal, or national level. A cell struggles for its own life and the life of cells that will issue from it. But it depends on the cells around it that support it and contribute to the existence of a livable environment.

Human beings have a drive to live for their own sake, each one of them. By the same token, human beings, by helping other people to live well and harmoniously, also create a favorable environment for themselves to thrive in. It may be enough, in order to contribute to the larger social organism of which each of us is a cell, merely to create favorable emotions within and around our own individual selves. This is surprisingly easy: just learn to be good to yourself.

In everyday life, and unless circumstances are exceptional, what is good is useful. It is often also profitable, and pleasant, and natural, and usually legal too. Every pleasure is good, unless it harms either yourself or others. To eat well, to make love well, to enjoy music, to enjoy nature, to avoid pain is good for you unless *you* know it's bad for you. It may seem ludicrous to state in all seriousness such an evident fact. But it is not when one sees the extent to which such evident truths are ignored.

The positive is what corresponds to essential, natural tendencies. It is made of feelings, thoughts, acts, that contribute to the improvement, the elevation of the individual — body and soul. Enthusiasm, hope, love, purposefulness, harmonious activity, satisfaction with one's accomplishments, mental and physical exercise, are positive. They bring no abnormal stresses that erode our vitality. They are all expressed in the most healthful of all states — that of joy.

Joy: The Gift You Give Yourself

If I were to recommend one single revitalization therapy, joy would be it. A man, however diminished, can draw from joy immense resources of vitality, and live a life fuller, more active, and more fruitful than the life of a man who enjoys perfect organic health but does not have the gift of joy. One of the most remarkable men I ever knew proved this to me beyond the shadow of a doubt.

I have already mentioned Ranko Kovljanic, and what he taught me about medicine. He also taught me about the power of the spirit.

My father had told me a story about Ranko many times. The two had met at the university in Budapest. Ranko had been a poor scholarship medical student and my father was from a wealthy family, but they became close friends. Ranko never allowed their differences in means to come between them in any way, and in fact Ranko never allowed my father to offer him money, and made it clear that he would refuse it had it been offered. In great difficulties, he persisted and managed to finish his medical degree.

The story my father told was that several years after he had graduated and returned to Belgrade, Ranko, who was still pursuing advanced studies, sent him an urgent telegram asking for a sizable loan. My father was surprised but he wired the money immediately. When he next saw Ranko some time later, the loan was never mentioned, although a few years later, my father suddenly began receiving payments with interest and within a short period the loan was paid off. This dignity and pride on Ranko's part greatly impressed my father.

One day when I was visiting Ranko the mysterious loan came into the conversation. I asked Ranko what it had been for. He told me that a student friend of his had come to him, distraught, one night and confessed that he had taken a lot of money from the student fund of which he was treasurer, and gambled it away. He planned to commit suicide, and wanted Ranko to tell the university authorities that he had paid for the theft with his life, but to see that his parents were told he had died in an accident.

Ranko simply wired my father for the money and replaced it. His friend didn't commit suicide, but continued medical school. Ranko went into the army and lost track of the fellow, who never repaid him. Eventually, Ranko paid my father back on his own.

Out of curiosity, I asked Ranko the man's name, and when he told me I immediately recognized the man as a highly successful Belgrade doctor. I explained that he had spent several years in the United States after he received his medical degree.

Ranko was delighted. He had started a foundation for blind physicians (since he felt that nothing was worse than blindness), and he promptly calculated that the sum due from the physician, including the interest of twenty years, would make a tidy contribution to it. He wrote to the man immediately, and a few days later came the reply — not from the wealthy doctor, but from his attorney. To this day, I remember the letter:

"Sir,
My client has advised me of the claim you have made. Would you please forward to me any material evidence substantiating it. May I point out that even if there is such evidence, a debt cannot be legally held if it has remained unclaimed for more than 10 years."

I raged. Ranko seemed undisturbed. "You know, I should have known better. I should have realized that if the man started by taking the money dishonestly he would be equally capable of refusing to repay me."

I wanted to leave for Belgrade immediately, to find the man and choke the money out of him — to expose the story and try to damage his career.

Ranko just smiled. Perhaps his wisdom told him there was no use in feeling revenge or hate. His world was positive, and perhaps he just didn't want negative feelings to interfere with it. He rolled his wheelchair over to the shelf where he kept his violin. He took it down — he played beautifully — and told me to take up mine, which I had with me. "Let's play some Bach," he said. "You'll see, everything will look different."

Of all the many things I learned from Ranko perhaps the most important was the power of true joy of the spirit. It is *a gift you give yourself* and one that is most valuable in times of difficult and stressful circumstances. It is the joy that corresponds to something that is right, natural, full of life. I don't know whether it is a sin to hate someone — if it is, I have occasionally been sinful — but it is harmful, sometimes more to the hater than the hated.

I have told the story of Ranko Kovljanic because he is, to me, an outstanding example of a man whose spirit had helped him not only overcome adversity, but find happiness in spite of it. The vitality he possessed, in spite of his physical handicaps, was exceptional. This is something science cannot explain, but something that is essential to the understanding of man, of his problems, of his diseases.

Aside from any ethical consideration, love is a basic need — to give love and to receive it. It is constructive, and it is therapeutic. Hostility is a disruptive emotion. How literally true is the expression, "There is bad blood between them."

The difference between the positive and the negative is instinctively known, it is built into us, because it is in relation to us that something beautiful is beautiful, and something ugly is ugly. And we know, instinctively as well as rationally, that the positive has a positive influence.

Finding Joy

Joy is the most effective, the most natural, the least expensive medicine, and it never has any harmful side effects. It is, however, habit forming, but I wouldn't worry about that.

Where do you find it? Certainly not in little boxes lined up on drugstore shelves. Look for it everywhere around you, and if you have trouble finding it, remember that joy, too, has a potent feedback effect. The more you give, the more you receive. And this is the most useful hint on how to go about finding joy for yourself: be a good egotist and start by giving joy to others. Sometimes it is the easiest way to start when you don't know how to give it to yourself. Then, wait and see it come bouncing back at you.

Part III: Revitalizing Techniques That Can Work

9. Live Foods:
From Steak Tartar to Nuts

Some people like to gamble, but nobody likes to lose. And certainly, nobody likes a game in which he doesn't have at least a chance to win.

This is why I don't try to compete with nature, since I am sure she can always do better. I have found it more rewarding to enlist her as my ally, maintaining a partnership that has existed for millions of years. Unfortunately, this is not universally the case. Civilized man often enters into competition with nature in the vain hope of improving on her.

Let's start with one example: All animals, except human beings and their domesticated animals, leap on their prey and eat it half alive, or else they eat fresh, live fruit or grass or roots.

Even a scavenger who eats carrion finds a lot of insect and bacteriological life crawling around in his cadavers. Civilized man, on the other hand, sterilizes, cooks, pasteurizes, and eats products into which chemicals are added to stop bacteriologic life.

We, civilized man, are missing something in our food: life. Although we do occasionally eat fresh fruits and vegetables, they are usually grown commercially, under the most perfect conditions, with the adjunct of chemical fertilizers and pesticides. They too are missing something: They have never struggled for life.

The nineteenth-century Russian scientist Vladimir Filatov found that living cells subjected to stress or fighting for survival produce biostimulins, short-lived substances that have long-lived effects in promoting survival. Like life itself, biostimulins have no known chemical formula, and cannot be synthesized.

Several years ago in the south of France, I inadvertently reaffirmed the truth of Filatov's theory of biostimulins. I had purchased some tomato plants, and, in the afternoon, the gardener planted some in a row. They promptly wilted and fell to the ground.

"Why haven't you watered them?" I asked.

"It's much better to water them in the evening," he said.

"That's silly. Let's plant another row and water it, and then we'll compare.

We did. Two days later, tomato plants in the row we had watered right after planting looked healthy and thriving. In the other row, one quarter of the plants had died.

"You see," I said, "I was right. We should have watered all of them."

"If you really want to know, let us compare the crop," answered the gardener.

A few months later, I found that the first row, which we had not watered right away and which had lost one quarter of its plants, gave not only a larger crop than the second but a tastier one too.

It was only later that I found out that Filatov, too, had experimented with plants and had come to the same conclusion as my gardener. We now use the principle of biostimulins in embryotherapy, described in Chapter 19.

Plants are no more made to live under glass than is man. They have, like man, the built-in potential for adaptation to the ups and downs of nature. They should, like man, be given a chance to struggle in order to grow stronger. But civilized man has created an atmosphere in which this struggle has been eliminated. From hothouse tomatoes (with their cottony texture and complete lack of flavor) to fodder-fed and steroid-fattened livestock and poultry, the food that comes to our tables has been practically nursed to death. And if we find these morsels not tender or tasty enough, we add meat tenderizers and MSG to amplify what little flavor remains.

Cooked Food is Dead Food

Cooking was the first major alteration in man's ancestral diet. Other, more recent, changes have been the preserving, canning, and freezing of food, as well as the introduction of new methods of producing food: chemical fertilizers and pesticides for fruit and vegetables, hormones and antibiotics for treatment of the animals we raise to eat.

A classical experiment illustrates the profound effect that the mere substitution of cooked meat for raw can have on the body. It was carried out more than 25 years ago by Dr. Francis M. Pottenger, Jr., who wanted to find out the effect of diet on the development of teeth. This he did, but he also learned quite a great deal more.

The experiment lasted several years, and nine hundred cats were used for it. The test was simple. Some of the cats were fed a diet consisting of two parts raw meat, one part raw milk, and some cod liver oil. The other cats received exactly the same diet, except that the meat was cooked.

The first group of cats reproduced normally from one generation to the next. Spontaneous abortion was rare, and the mother cats nursed their young normally. The cats had good resistance to infection and exhibited a pleasant disposition.

For the second group, I'd like to quote the results, published by Dr. Pottenger in the *American Journal of Orthodontics and Oral Surgery.*

> [*These*] *cats . . . reproduced a heterogeneous strain of kittens, each kitten of the litter being different in skeletal pattern. Abortion in these cats was common, running about 25 per cent in the first generation to about 70 per cent in the second generation. Deliveries were in general difficult, many cats dying in labor. Mortality rates of the kittens were high, frequently due to the failure of the mother to lactate. . . . At times the mother would steadily decline in health following the birth of the kittens, dying from some obscure tissue exhaustion about three months after delivery. Others experienced increasing difficulty with subsequent pregnancies. Some failed to become pregnant. . . .*
>
> [*The*] *cats were irritable. . . . Sex interest was slack or perverted. Vermin and intestinal parasites abounded. Skin lesions and allergies were frequent, being progressively worse from one generation to the next. Pneumonia and empyema were among the principal causes of natural death among the adult cats. Diarrhea, followed by pneumonia, took a heavy toll of the kittens. Osteomyelitis, hepatitis, orchitis, oophoritis, paralysis, meningitis, cystitis, arthritis, and many other degenerative lesions familiar in human medicine were observed.*
>
> *Of the cats maintained entirely on the cooked-meat diet, with raw milk, the kittens of the third generation were so degenerated that none of them survived the sixth month of life,* thereby terminating the strain. (*Emphasis mine.*)

Similar effects have been observed in people, notably in primitive communities living on the fringes of civilization and exposed to civilized food previously not known to them.

If I had the opportunity of making only one recommendation with regard to food, it would be the following: You should be careful not only of what you eat but of what you don't eat.

Everything that we need is in nature, otherwise we wouldn't be here discussing it. Mankind evolved without synthetic vitamins, food additives, or enriched meals. If something goes wrong now, it is largely because we have *subtracted from nature*. We talk of enzymes, biostimulins, trace elements, and vitamins. If they are missing in our food, it is because we've done something to the food or not taken advantage of all that nature has put at our disposal. Aside from the folly of trying to restore those vital elements we have removed by processing, there is also the futility of such an effort. We cannot put everything back because we don't know everything that we have taken out.

Some of the alterations to which food is subjected during cooking, canning, and freezing are known. Foods to be canned or frozen are first blanched either by immersion in hot water or by spraying with steam. This kills any possible bacteria, but also kills the life in the food — that is, if you plant it afterwards, it will not grow. Cooking, canning, and freezing also destroy some vitamins and enzymes. Vitamin C is particularly sensitive to heat and cannot survive the blanching process. A large proportion of vitamin B_6, pantothenic acid, folic acid, and biotin are also lost and are not reintroduced into food during enrichment. Vitamins B_1, B_2, and niacin, however, are sometimes added.

After blanching, canned foods are once more exposed to hot water and steam, while food to be frozen goes directly to the rapid-freezer. Only certain fruits are not blanched but instead are preserved in sugar syrup and some chemicals to prevent oxidation. Freezing is less destructive than heat, so, as a rule, frozen food loses less of its vital elements than does canned food.

It is known that the modern diet of processed, cooked food is associated with dental cavities, skeletal defects, fatigue, and a number of degenerative diseases. But our organism is very resistant to illness and adaptive to change. Bad feeding habits can exist for years before they provoke serious diseases. Very often, these diseases can be cured amazingly fast by returning to an adequate diet.

Our consumption of impoverished and biologically transformed products of nature is inevitable, and we have to cope with it. We should be conscious of the amount of refined food we eat. In fifty years, fat consumption has gone up 50 percent, but sugar consumption has gone up 500 percent. And we should balance our diet with at least some of the live elements man has ingested during countless generations.

Organic Food

One of the problems with fresh fruit and vegetables is the use of pesticides, insecticides, and artificial fertilizers by commercial growers. There has been a lot of talk about organic food in recent years, and it is evident that organically grown (i.e. without using chemicals) foods are better. But they are expensive and not always available. Worse, the success of organically grown foods has been such that "organic" foods aren't always organic. (Not long ago a California organic food grower was caught spraying his orchards and gardens at night.)

Fortunately, agricultural pesticides hardly ever penetrate beyond the skin of a fruit or vegetable, and there's the safe solution of peeling. On the other hand, the skin usually contains, weight for weight, many more nutritional elements and vitamins than does the pulp. Chemical fertilizers also deprive the product of some trace and nutritional elements available in good soil fertilized with manure. It is interesting to note that Europeans, who are not yet accustomed to the intensive use of agricultural chemicals, are usually disappointed by American fruits and vegetables because they have an attractive appearance and size but not much taste.

Organic food is fine, and it is a step toward nature, but we still cook too much of our food. Organic or not, we do need some raw natural foods in order to introduce at least some live elements into our organism. A small amount can make a big difference.

Professor Griffon's Wind-Drier

I make no secret of my preference for fresh, live food, but I also recognize that it is not always readily or economically available to everyone. I continue to hope that the modern scientific wizards will develop a method of conserving food without killing it and adulterating it to the extent that now seems necessary. One such process has been developed, but, for various reasons, it has not gained wide acceptance.

I am speaking of the process developed by Professor Henri Griffon, retired director of the Paris Laboratory of Toxicology and member of the French Academy of Pharmacy, who has been engaged in research as a member of the European Commission on Food Additives. In Europe alone, and even within the Common Market, there is no uniform legislation on additives, as there is none on pesticides and insecticides. Some food additives and preservatives widely used, for example, in Germany are considered harmful and are banned in France.

Griffon became preoccupied by the whole problem of food preservation, realizing that none of the currently used methods preserve the value of the produce being conserved. There is one technique that does it better than others, and that is lyophilization (dehydration at low temperature and under high vacuum, which we call freeze-drying), but it is too costly to be used as a standard method of food preservation.

Griffon felt that something should be done to avoid the daily damage and waste inflicted by most food-processing methods. He came upon a successful method of food preservation quite by accident. One rainy day, he saw his mother taking some wet washed laundry outdoors.

"What are you doing?" he asked her. "It's raining."

"I know," she answered. "But there's a good wind, too." And she hung the laundry to dry in an area protected from the rain but exposed to the wind. It dried rapidly.

Professor Griffon decided to try a similar drying process with food. He was not an engineer but insisted on designing his own wind-drier, into which he introduced a number of different ground-up foods. The food moved along a kind of roller system and was exposed to a fairly strong wind produced by an electric fan. It worked perfectly.

Meat, eggs, fruit, and vegetables, thus deprived of most but not all of their water content, can be preserved for months and well over a year, without canning or the use of any additives.

They have not been exposed to heat and so retain nearly all of their vitamins and other live elements. They are fundamentally unaltered and keep their taste.

When I visited Griffon's setup, some wind-dried food was stored away, simply placed in open sacks lined up on shelves. Griffon took a handful of eggs he had wind-dried two years earlier, and made an omelet. I wouldn't have been able to tell the difference from one made from fresh eggs.

I must say that when I saw the device he had put together, it looked like something that is referred to in America as a Rube Goldberg machine.

He patented his process and offered the patent to one or two food-processing companies. Specialists designed simplified machines that could be made for large-scale processing, and accountants calculated the cost of the process. It was, he was told, higher by 3 or 4 percent than other methods, and this, added to the cost of raw materials, administrative and advertising costs, would have reduced the profit margin or increased the sales price. Why take the risk, as long as people are satisfied with what they get, even if they don't know exactly what they get?

As far as I know, Griffon's wind-drier is still on the shelf, and so is some of the food he's dried in it.

What You Can Do To Improve Your Diet

But what, you may ask, can be done within the realm of practicable reality to improve your health and chances for a long life in terms of the food you eat?

I am not a food crank. I do not live on organic food, and I don't drink fresh blood. I enjoy smoked ham or tournedos Rossini with a good wine, and I don't recommend that we go to the forest at lunchtime to stalk our daily prey and sink our teeth into its throbbing flesh. In fact, as you'll remember from Chapter 5, I don't even recommend a specific diet. I usually mistrust articles and books that do this. Different people have different needs, and the best book for you would be one written especially for you, after a thorough study of your case.

I'm often asked by people who live in the city what they can do to come closer to nature, to find all of these essential life elements.

During my life and practice in several countries, I have learned a few things about food, and I think I can give a few useful hints. They will be hints; I shall prescribe no regimen nor will I recommend that you weigh your slices of bread. I don't expect that all the hints will be followed. Pick one, or two, or five, whatever is most suitable to you or seems most attractive or feasible.

Many such hints I learned from Ranko, my old Yugoslav mentor. Ranko had made a study of the local folk medicine, which, he had found, maintained most of the local population in excellent health and helped it reach longevity that was exceptional by urban standards.

He collected and tested the various foods, herbs, leaves, and roots used by the Serbs and their Bulgarian neighbors. He then used, with excellent results, some of this "medicine" on his urban patients.

Folk medicine may rely partly on legend and partly on the belief that it does wonders, but it is known today that nature holds the secrets of many potent medicines. No single drug, no single plant or natural food either is a panacea. But the associated action of several natural elements can have a striking revitalizing effect.

Some Basic Live Foods

Little things make big differences. A small amount of live food acts as a catalyst. You can, for instance, eat live oysters or clams — even one or two will help. You can eat yogurt, and all fermented cheeses. Fermented cheeses like Camembert, Brie, Roquefort, and the various "blue" cheeses are full of life. In fact, you have doubtless enjoyed many of the foods described here without realizing they were live.

Soybeans

Another valuable live food is soybean sprouts. The secret of soybean sprouts is an enzyme called invertase. This enzyme, which is not available on the market in its pure form and is not used as a food additive because of its high cost, can be grown in your own kitchen. Simply cover the bottom of a bowl or plate with damp cotton, gauze, or a clean cloth. Spread some soybeans on top and keep your garden moist by watering lightly now and then. Within a few days the beans will sprout. When they have grown about an inch and a half long and the tops have turned green, harvest the crop by plucking them from the cotton and removing the roots. The entire sprout can be eaten raw and used in any way that you would normally use a salad green.

Invertase is an essential enzyme because it helps convert poly-saccharides and disaccharides into monosaccharides, the only carbohydrate that can be directly assimilated by the human body. The high invertase content of soybeans was discovered by the French during their military involvement in Vietnam. Amazed at the capacity of the Viet Minh to survive on an almost exclusively carbohydrate diet, French doctors reproduced their eating habits under laboratory conditions. The presence of soybean sprouts was noted, and, upon analysis, invertase was discovered to be present in significant quantities. The Viet Minh, however unwittingly, were providing themselves with a living factor which converted their otherwise impoverished diet into one that gave the body a large amount of easily convertible energy.

With young soybean sprouts snipped from your 10-inch home garden, you will get, in addition to invertase, natural protein, lecithin, biostimulins and trephones, a growth factor described in Chapter 17.

Fresh, raw fruits and vegetables
So far, there is no widespread method of preserving all of the value of fruits and vegetables to make them available out of season or away from the production area. The canned products can never be as good as the fresh. Even if the label insists there are no *additives*, you can be sure there are *subtractives*, usually the result of denaturations by heat. Fortunately, fresh fruit and vegetable juices are becoming increasingly available, but whole fruits and vegetables are better. And I mean whole: skin and

seeds included. Seeds are the fruits' eggs or embryos; they contain nutritive and vital elements absent from the juice and pulp. I do not mean that you should try to swallow avocado pits or choke on whole apricots and peaches, but with such fruits as grapes, apples, pears, and berries, the seeds may be eaten with ease.

If you have a small garden, it's fine to have flowers, but why not plant, in between, a few radishes, carrots, a salad? To those who live in the city, I often say that a patch of ground the size of a desk is enough to supplement a person's diet with a minimum live food requirement. Or else, if you have a dry storage place, keep apples, apricots, mushrooms, that can all be conserved for months without undergoing destructive blanching and the eventual addition of artificial flavor. If you have access to organic food, I would recommend particularly those you eat raw, of which you eat the skin. In apples, tomatoes, pears, and some other fruits, there are more vitamins in the skin and just underneath it than there are on the inside. The same applies to outer leaves of salad greens and cabbage, and it makes sense to buy organic fruits and vegetables if only to make sure that pesticides haven't penetrated into the outer skin.

Juices are particularly recommended. You should try (and I would say at almost any cost, and certainly at the cost of a fruit juicer) to prevent your children's becoming addicted to pops and cola drinks, whether carbonated or not. It is so widely known that these damage teeth and the digestive system that I am amazed that they are still so abundantly available to youngsters of the civilized world (even the Russians have taken to cola drinks lately). Fresh fruit and vegetable juices, aside from being health-giving, are among the most effective means to avoid this juvenile addiction.

And I insist on fresh juices. Canned fruits and canned juices are certainly less harmful than soda drinks, and some of them are even good for you, but vitamins and other vital elements have been mercilessly exterminated by heat. Canned fruits are a different matter; sometimes they are not blanched but preserved in sugar syrup. The syrup usually contains some of the vitamins that would have been lost through heating, but if you are to take

advantage of these, you also have to take the dubious advantage
of the added sugar.

Yogurt

Another important live food is yogurt. Highly digestible, an
excellent source of protein, and available in fat-free form, yogurt
is a live, entirely natural food.

Yogurt is made by introducing into heated milk one of a few
strains of bacteria, notably *Lactobacillus bulgaricus* (the name indicates the Balkan origin, although yogurt, under slightly different forms, has long been known in many other countries). The
milk is then kept warm, approximately at body temperature, for
several hours, while the bacteria reproduce, thicken the milk,
and give it its unmistakable taste.

The bacteria, not only harmless but beneficial, remain alive,
and the two most important nutrients in milk, calcium and protein, remain intact. *Lactobacillus bulgaricus* closely resembles *Lactobacillus bifidus*, which makes up the intestinal flora of an infant
who lives exclusively on mother's milk.

Yogurt can be easily made at home, providing a cheaper and
fresher supply of this important food than is available at your
local supermarket. There are a number of yogurt makers available, but even if you don't have one you can produce a creamy
and delicious yogurt in your kitchen. Simply add a tablespoon
of yogurt culture (available as such in health food stores, though
you can also use the same amount from existing yogurt) to a
quart of milk which has been heated just to body temperature.
That's all — no gelatin, no preservatives, no additives of any
sort. Place this mixture in a clean glass container and leave it in a
warm and quiet place for eight to twelve hours. The longer it is
kept at room temperature, the tangier it will be.

The most important things to remember about making yogurt
are that warmth (not heat) and absolute stillness are required. A
proper temperature can be maintained by placing your cultured
milk near the stove, in an elevated spot away from drafts, or in
an unheated oven. If your oven has a pilot light it will ensure an
evenly moderate temperature during the time the yogurt is incubating. You can protect the yogurt from vibration by making it

overnight when activity in the kitchen is at a minimum. Otherwise the container may be cushioned in a box lined with foam rubber. (The commercial yogurt makers are essentially nothing more than such a cushioned box with a low-level heating element provided.) Once you've started your own yogurt culture, simply remember to keep a tablespoon from the last batch with which to make the next one.

Any milk can be used to make yogurt. In Bulgaria and Serbia, yogurt is made with cow, buffalo, sheep, or goat milk. In Russia, mare's milk is also used. Delicious yogurt can even be made with nonfat dried milk, though of course the richest, most vital yogurt is made from unpasteurized whole milk.

Buy or make plain yogurt, free of artificial flavorings and preserves. If you don't like the taste, add some natural flavoring yourself: fresh fruits or honey, or even salt and pepper.

Claims of the therapeutic value of yogurt date back to the beginning of history, but the first thorough study was made by Professor Elie Metchnikoff, one of Pasteur's earliest collaborators, who later received the Nobel Prize for the discovery of phagocytes, our bodies' front-line defense system of white blood cells.

Metchnikoff was also one of the first gerontologists. He maintained that death was not a normal physiologic phenomenon but a chronic disease, against which a remedy could theoretically be found. Gerontology would have progressed more rapidly if Metchnikoff's contributions hadn't been forgotten for a time and later rediscovered. Ironically, he is best remembered as a promoter of yogurt, which he was. He is also said to have called yogurt the elixir of life, which he didn't.

He knew that in many Bulgarian villages an unusually large proportion of people lived to be more than 100 years old. As a youth in Russia, Metchnikoff had often eaten yogurt, and as a bacteriologist at the Pasteur Institute he was interested in finding out just what happened when milk turned sour.

He isolated *Lactobacillus bulgaricus* in his laboratory and recommended it as an antidote against intoxication by other bacteria. Some of his conclusions were confirmed by research in American hospitals, where it was shown that *L. acidophilus* improved bowel function and acted favorably against digestive tract diseases, such as constipation, colitis, and ulcers.

What Metchnikoff believed — and I have found it to be true — is though yogurt is not *the* elixir of life, it is *one* of the foods of longevity. There is not one food staple, one drug, one treatment, one beverage, that will prolong life appreciably. Aging is a widespread degenerative disease that cannot be treated by a single therapeutic agent but by a multitherapeutic approach. Yogurt is part of this approach.

It has been found effective in curing digestive illnesses caused by the too frequent use of antibiotics which often results in the destruction of intestinal flora. Professor René Dubos, of the Rockefeller University, has found that yogurt also increases resistance to infection and prolongs the life span of animals.

The current yogurt fashion in America is, indeed, to be welcomed. It has followed by a few years a similar phenomenon in Europe, where many physicians and nutritionists have confirmed that yogurt is a healthy and tasty live food.

Raw steak (or steak tartar)

Freshly ground raw steak, prepared with chopped raw chive or onion, oil, pepper, and other ingredients to your taste, is excellent. Most people say they don't like it even before trying it, yet all the meat we once ate was raw. To make sure the meat is freshly ground, select your own piece, with little or no fat in it, and have it ground in front of you in a clean grinder (one not used for pork), or do it at home. (To be on the safe side, pregnant women should avoid raw steak, as food poisoning can precipitate toxemia of pregnancy.)

Garlic

This is not only live food but an excellent, natural antiseptic that has been shown to decrease the number of dangerous bacteria in the digestive tract. Garlic medicines exist in capsule form. They have antiseptic properties but obviously not all of the qualities of fresh raw garlic. It is unfortunate that in much of the civilized world (not all of it) garlic and other members of the onion family are considered to have an antisocial, unpleasant smell. This can be avoided to a great extent by mixing garlic with fresh parsley, or even better, by chewing fresh parsley or a few roasted coffee beans after the meal. (Parsley has the advantage over chlorophyll chewing gum of containing not sugar and synthetic colorants but, instead, a large amount of vitamins.)

So ancient is the belief in garlic's qualities that it is related to history's first known labor strikes, some 5,000 years ago. The slaves building the Cheops pyramid refused to work when their daily ration of garlic was curtailed. Now even the scientifically inclined recognize the value of garlic, because they have identified in it at least one active bactericidal substance, called allyl disulfate. It makes up only a very small part of garlic, but it's the part that smells. It is also worth noting that the regular use of garlic by people with hypertension has been associated with reduced blood pressure.

Honey and pollen

Another food, known since time immemorial for its therapeutic qualities, is honey. The "nectar of the Gods" was long accepted as a beneficial gift of nature, but today the scientist, who does not like mysteries, has been able to explain some of the benefits provided by honey.

Honey is made from pollen, the male germ seed of plants, flowers, or tree blossoms. This pollen is collected on the bees' hairy legs, taken to the hive, and mixed with nectar, the sweet substance of flowers that the bees swallow and then disgorge for honey-making.

Each plant produces a different kind of pollen, each containing different amounts and kinds of vitamins, minerals, and other substances that have not yet been identified. Bees like organic food, the cranks! Experiments have shown that, given the choice between a field treated with chemicals and an untreated one, bees invariably start for the latter.

Honey is a good medium for preserving vitamins. It also contains copper, iron, calcium, sodium, magnesium, manganese, phosphorus, silicon, sulfur, titanium, and potassium, trace elements required by the body in very small amounts. Pollen — and honey — also contain amino acids, the building blocks that make up protein. Of the more than twenty important amino acids that are known to occur naturally, the human body can synthesize about half. Those we can't manufacture are called "essential amino acids." Since we can't make them, they must come with our food. Ten amino acids are considered essential to adults, eleven to children, and honey contains all of them.

Honey also contains, of course, sugar, but not the complex sugars found in cane sugar or starches. These sugars must undergo enzymatic breakdown in the digestive tract and colon to be changed into simple sugars that can be assimilated. In honey, this work has already been done by the bee. This is particularly useful when one needs a quick supply of sugar energy, has a weak digestion, or cannot, for some reason, make the conversion.

Pollen and honey also contain an antibiotic that is capable of destroying or weakening some pathologic microorganisms, such as those of typhoid fever, dysentery, and bacteria associated with bronchopneumonia, peritonitis, and suppurative abscesses. This has been clearly demonstrated simply by placing honey into cultures of these microorganisms. French researchers have also found recently that honey contains a growth factor that acts as a tonic and seems to produce an improvement in general health. Anemia in children should always be investigated by a doctor as to its cause, but in my experience I have found that anemic children, regularly given honey, almost invariably show an increase in red corpuscles.

Aside from being the best natural sweetener known, nonirritative of the digestive tract, a live food containing natural vitamins, minerals, and growth factors, I have found the following properties of honey particularly useful.

It has a gentle laxative effect and can overcome chronic constipation even when other remedies fail. At the same time, it helps treat other intestinal conditions, including diarrhea. This is not contradictory. As a natural remedy it tends to regularize the functions of the intestine, bringing them toward the norm.

It is a mild sedative. Accompanied by a proper relaxation technique, the taking of honey in the evening can induce sleep that is natural and that should be undisturbed. Like anything in nature, the results are never 100 percent. For some people, depending on the cause of their insomnia, honey will not work. Others may require a single teaspoonful of honey in the evening, and still others may need three before drowsiness sets in. This sedative action is also useful in case of a cough. To help clear the bronchial passages, it is better to mix lemon with honey and drink the mixture warm.

Honey can also be used topically, to help the healing of wounds. Not long ago it was found to be particularly effective against bed sores, which are sometimes resistant to all other forms of treatment.

Unfortunately, there is a tendency these days to cook honey before putting it into jars, so that it stays clear and does not harden. This destroys some of its properties. Hardened honey is excellent and tasty, and some people prefer it. Otherwise it is enough to place the honey jar in warm water (not excessively hot) to clear and liquefy it. Honey straight from the hive, centrifuged with some of the dust in the hive, is even better. The dust is nothing but pollen.

Pollen in itself is sometimes used in tablet form. Most of the recent studies about pollen have been carried out in Sweden (the pollen is collected by pollen traps set up at the entrance of beehives; some of the pollen carried by the bee is brushed off its legs and collected). Natural pollen extracts — cernitin — contain all of the known amino acids, all of the known vitamins, trace elements, and even some hormones. In other words, they contain many of the elements essential to life.

In tests carried out in Europe and in America, pollen was proven to be an excellent body-builder, and it is used by athletes during the Olympic games. Some physicians recommend "pollen courses" — the taking of pollen as a daily food supplement for a given period.

Grape cures

I have found that honey courses, or cures, are excellent, and the same, I suppose, applies for pollen. Cures of fruits and vegetables of the season are traditionally used in many countries, and they help eliminate toxins that accumulate in the body. A grape cure in the fall, for four or five days such as described in a weight-reducing regimen in Chapter 5, is an excellent purifier. You can also do this in winter or spring or whenever you can get fresh grapes of any kind.

Grapes should be washed well but eaten with the skin and with the seeds as well. (Washing is more efficient when the grapes have been removed from the stalks.) The seeds are the grape's embryos, and even if they are not completely digested, they do no harm and may release during their journey some of their essential elements. I have no proof for this, but it seems logical, and there's no risk in trying.

During a grape cure one may, of course, eat other food, but keep the emphasis on grapes and avoid proteins (replacing them with carbohydrates, such as spaghetti, if you need something to fill you up) so as not to interfere with detoxification.

If you live in apple country, try the apple cure or a cure associating two or three vegetables. During these cures, it is a good idea to drink about a quart of water a day. It will help eliminate the toxins that break away when you start utilizing some of your storage tissues.

Apple cider vinegar

The drinking of two teaspoonfuls of apple cider vinegar, diluted in a glass of water, every morning, has a general tonifying effect and can even be useful in the treatment of some forms of obesity. It is also a healing agent and an antiseptic, thus useful also in the treatment of menstrual troubles, hemorrhages such as nose bleeding, and superficial cuts. It has been traditionally said that cider vinegar "dries up the blood," and the results obtained confirm that there is truth in this belief. During such treatments, larger doses can be taken for a few days — up to four or five glasses of the diluted solution.

Yeast

This is a very important live food. It contains *all* of the B vitamins in their natural form. Yeast is actually a living plant, a tiny fungus about one five-thousandth of an inch in diameter, which is grown commercially in vats under precisely controlled conditions. When the growth of yeast stops because there's no more food to grow from and no more room for yeast to grow, the waste products are discarded, and the yeast can be preserved, either alive in cake form or dried in tablet or powder form.

There are several types of yeast (wine ferments, thanks to yeast, and the great French vineyards boast of their own variety, which accounts in part for the quality of wine), but the two most easily available commercially are brewer's yeast and baker's yeast. Both contain appreciable amounts of B vitamins and also protein. Some companies grow yeast especially as food supplement, adding this or that to the culture medium to increase the nutrient value or food content of yeast.

All of these are fine, and yeast found in health stores does give you the wide spectrum vitamin B complex. The only shortcoming is that it is dead yeast. Once you have realized the benefit of live food, it is understandable that you should seek live yeast. Live, solid yeast can be found in food markets and in old-fashioned bakeries. It is a solid mass, best kept under refrigeration, and known as "cake-form" yeast. You don't have to chew it. If you add a little salt and stir with a spoon, it becomes liquid within seconds. You can drink it after mixing it with a little water, but if you don't like the taste, add some beer instead. It blends very well with it.

Some people have said that live yeast should never be eaten, because it also consumes B vitamins, and should it survive within you, it will take away the vitamins. This argument has only one redeeming quality: it is amusing. I can imagine (although to my knowledge it hasn't been tried) that a man thrown into a vatful of yeast might, indeed, yield some vitamins to the tiny fungi. But when a spoonful of yeast is ingested, the odds are overwhelmingly in your favor: You'll eat the yeast, it won't eat you. Don't worry about cake-form live yeast, but imagine, instead, that you might be getting some additional benefits, as you do when you swallow any live food, particularly when it has growth potential. Why take synthetic B vitamin pills, when one cent's worth of yeast gives you the assurance of providing you with the whole spectrum of these vitamins, perhaps including some that have not yet been isolated.

Wheat germ

Wheat germ is a healthy, live food that contains a lot of vitamin E. Until a few decades ago, wheat germ was found in many wheat products. However, because it is particularly perishable, most packagers of wheat products began to remove the wheat germ to increase the shelf life of their goods, and at the present time, the germ is absent from nearly all standard cereal products. We are thus deprived of something that once was part of our normal diet. However, you can buy it and store it in the refrigerator for a certain time.

The best way to eat wheat germ is raw. If you don't like the taste, toast it lightly. But remember that toasting eliminates the heat-sensitive vitamins, and of course you kill the wheat germ itself. It is better to use it raw in salads, as part of the dressing, where its taste blends with others. Plain yogurt with fresh wheat germ and some honey for sweetening is a particularly tasty and vital combination. I have been informed that the Soviet cosmonauts eat it for breakfast.

A word of caution about wheat germ *oil*. Good wheat germ oil tends to become rancid fairly rapidly. It loses its effectiveness and then has a negative effect, as does any rancid oil. Even when it is fresh, wheat germ oil simply does not contain all the elements contained in wheat germ.

Other natural products

Some other live foods and natural products also have very precise physiologic effects. (Plants and their therapeutic effects are discussed in Chapter 11.)

Cherries are a laxative, and an infusion made with *cherry stems* is an excellent diuretic. During the cherry season every spring, the Serbian peasants take a diuretic cure that has become traditional. Such a periodic treatment can eliminate toxins that may have accumulated, even if their effects are not yet apparent.

Watermelon, too, has a similar action. Ranko Kovljanic told me of one of his patients who had bladder stones. After their painful elimination, the man kept the stones on the table of his dining room as a vivid reminder that he should not eat too much.

One day he was eating a watermelon, and some juice ran over the symbolic bladder stones; to his amazement, the stones were corroded and almost dissolved by the juice.

Nuts (not canned nor in plastic bags) and fresh *parsley* can easily be found. The so-called virgin *olive oil,* obtained by first extraction (not by heat or chemical solvents but by pressure), is available in health food and some luxury stores. *Sauerkraut* is excellent live food, not the canned kind but the fermented cabbage such as is sold right out of the barrel in many delicatessen stores.

I have tried, in the course of this chapter, to give you some hints to help you increase the proportion of live, natural foods in your diet. If you gradually introduce these elements into your daily routine, you will find that, almost without effort, you have enriched your own vitality. In closing I would like to leave you with this bit of advice: in general, choose whole foods rather than segments of food. Whole wheat flour, for instance, is preferable to white flour. White flour does not contain wheat germ, which is the grain's embryo and which also contains a much larger concentration of protein. The starchy white flour, of course, is often said to be "enriched," but the process of impoverishing food by subtracting some vital elements from it, and then enriching it by adding other elements considered to be good, is utter nonsense. It is conceit to feel we can do better than nature, particularly when we don't know precisely what it is we remove from food during treatment.

10. Vitamins, Enzymes, and Trace Elements

One day I gave a talk about vitamins and trace elements at a British university, and a man asked to see me after the conference. He had, he said, a peculiar vitamin problem and started explaining to me some of the vitamin deficiencies he was suffering from.

I saw him again on the following day. He was an accountant in his 30's and a very methodical man. He brought along a list of the pills he was taking. There were 27 of them.

He had been disappointed with his physician and had started reading everything available about vitamins. All the pills he was taking were available over the counter and had been self-prescribed. Fourteen of them contained various elements of the

B vitamin complex, some with other vitamins and vitamin associations, others with trace metals.

I proposed giving him one preparation to replace all he was taking. The prescription, I told him, would be prepared especially for him. In fact, it was a placebo (I don't remember exactly what it was, perhaps just water colored with tea), and he took it faithfully for a fortnight.

When I saw him again, it was obvious that he did have a vitamin deficiency, and the symptoms of nervousness and bad memory indicated that it was in the B group. I replaced the placebo drug with yeast — nothing but live yeast, to be taken three times a week.

My patient knew nothing about yeast. It is, by and large, ignored by medical writers, and its use is not encouraged by the pharmaceutical industry, most likely because it is too easy to make. It doesn't pay to advertise because it can't be patented, and it is inexpensive.

His subjective symptoms rapidly disappeared. There was no doubt that this was the result of yeast treatment rather than the placebo effect resulting from belief in the treatment. I explained to him that yeast contained all of the vitamin B complex and outlined the effects of vitamin B deficiency. I think he resented a bit the method I had employed to detoxicate him from his pill addiction, but the resentment didn't last long.

Vitamins

Of course he, like everybody else, had heard of vitamins. And, like almost everybody, he was full of misconceptions about them. Vitamins are regulatory substances, catalysts, which are needed in very small quantities — a human body contains about one fourth of an ounce of vitamin compounds. Avitaminosis, the deficiency disease due to lack of vitamins, is very seldom seen in advanced societies, as most of us get a sufficient supply of vitamins in our food. Massive overdoses of certain vitamins, however, can lead to disease and create an unnatural adaptation: a drug dependence such that the return to a normal absorption may lead to a withdrawal situation that can be compared to a self-induced deficiency. Particularly dangerous are overdoses of the fat-soluble vitamins, notably A and D, which are found dissolved in the fats of food like butter and egg yolk. This type of vitamin is stored and accumulated by the body, and the toxicity of overdoses has long been proven.

Vitamin A

This vitamin is necessary to overall vision, growth, and bone development in young people, to the formation of teeth, and to the health of tissues lining our bodies. It is present in milk, cream, cheeses, butter, and meat (particularly liver) and can be formed from carotene, a vitamin precursor found in vegetables. Vitamin A, in other words, is plentiful in a normal diet, and supplements should be taken only on prescription, when vitamin A deficiency has been established. Overdoses can provoke extreme fatigue, anemia, mouth ulcers, cracking of the skin, and a condition known as pseudotumor cerebri — a buildup of pressure in the head that mimics a brain tumor. Overdosage is particularly dangerous in children: it can provoke structural bone changes and physical stunting. There is evidence that overdoses can also cause menstrual irregularities, insomnia, and mental complications.

However, Max Wolf, a patriarch of American gerontology, in collaboration with several German scientists, has been experimenting on the use of high, nearly toxic dosages of Vitamin A, combined with enzymes, in the treatment of cancer. Very interesting results have been achieved in the prevention of metastasis and easing the painful terminal stages.

Vitamin B group

An important vitamin of the water-soluble group (which also includes vitamin C) is vitamin B or, rather, the vitamin B group (or complex). All of its members are related and tend to be found in the same foods (and all of them occur in yeast). It is important to remember that water-soluble vitamins are affected by cooking. Two of the most important members of this group are thiamine (or B_1), whose shortage can cause fatigue, irritability, mental disturbance, muscle cramps, and riboflavin (or B2), whose deficiency can cause tissue breakdown, making cracks at the corners of the mouth and giving bloodshot eyes. Riboflavin can be destroyed by light: if a milk bottle is left outdoors for two hours, two thirds of its riboflavin content can be lost.

High dosages of B12 have been successfully used in the treatment of pernicious anemia, and lately John M. Ellis, M.D. and James Presley have suggested high dosages of Vitamin B6 can be used in the treatment of arthritic conditions.

Vitamin C

There is an ongoing controversy about vitamin C, concerning, among other things, its protective action against the common cold. I think the controversy can be settled by recognizing that vitamin C cannot be made by or stored in the human body and is extremely perishable, and because few of us receive enough of it in our daily diet, a supplement may be required. Though nearly all animal species manufacture vitamin C, ascorbic acid, in their own bodies, so far as is known, only man, other primates, the guinea pig, one species of Indian bat, and an Oriental bird are unable to manufacture this vital acid as needed. This lack, perhaps lost through an evolutionary accident, poses an intriguing question: Since we can't make it or store it in our tissues, how much should we take of it?

Research shows that the animals and insects that do manufacture vitamin C produce what amounts to a daily 15 grams for a 150-pound man. The gorilla who, like man, cannot manufacture vitamin C eats food in his natural habitat that supplies about 4.5 grams a day. Linus Pauling, the Nobel prize-winning chemist, has estimated that the raw, natural plants on which our ancestors lived provided 2.3 to 9 grams of vitamin C daily.

Although the 10 milligrams available in the daily food we eat may be sufficient to protect us against scurvy, Pauling has found it insufficient for the optimal functioning of cells and tissues. He recommends a daily dose at least fifty times as high — 500 milligrams.

Unless we return to the diet of primitive man, there's no way of getting this amount without taking supplementary vitamin C.

This will not insure a fifty-fold improvement of health, but it definitely helps. Clinical studies have shown that groups of people taking high doses of vitamin C have the common cold about half as often as people taking minimal doses.

This suggests that the usually recommended daily intakes are too low. The recommendations vary between 30 milligrams, according to the Canadian Dietary Standard for Adults a few years ago, to 60 and 75 milligrams for normal adults, according to the National Research Council of the U.S.A. More like 500 milligrams daily is required by man. If there seems to be an epidemic of colds, or if you are exposed to a high risk of contracting a cold, the dose can be doubled. Vitamin C is one of the least toxic substances: since it can't be stored in the body, any excess is passed almost immediately. The only possible side effect is that the urine becomes acidified. Pauling says this can be avoided by taking an antacid or, more simply, by taking not ascorbic acid but sodium ascorbate, marketed as "chewable vitamin C." Naturally vitamin C requirements vary from person to person. The specific requirement can be established through a urine saturation test, a laboratory procedure.

Vitamin C also seems to reduce cholesterol deposits in the arteriovascular system. This and other discoveries are among the fruits of extensive research which is being done on this mysterious but important vitamin.

Vitamin C requirements have special significance for women who take contraceptive pills. Not long ago British researcher Dr. Michael Briggs made a study of the breakdown and loss of vitamin C in the organism and found that the breakdown is speeded up during the absorption of estrogens. He observed that ascorbic acid levels in blood particles (leukocytes and platelets) were significantly lower in women taking sex hormone contraceptives than in women who either did not take the pill or were pregnant. This has been confirmed in animal experiments carried out by other researchers.

This breakdown seems accelerated by the stimulant action of the estrogens through the liver, and it seems possible some of the side effects of the pill may be a consequence of this vitamin shortage. So it may be helpful, and certainly won't be harmful, if women taking oral contraceptives get into the habit of downing the pill with a glass of orange juice. An orange three inches in diameter provides about 70 milligrams of vitamin C.

Vitamin D

Another vitally important vitamin is "the sunshine vitamin," vitamin D, which occurs naturally only in animals and in some decomposing plants exposed to ultraviolet radiation. Recent findings have revealed that this vitamin, in fact, operates like a hormone.

Vitamin D is part of the mechanism that maintains the correct balance of calcium in the body. Calcium is needed not only for bone formation but for nerve function and many enzymatic reactions. Several substances are involved in calcium metabolism: a substance known as calcitonin reduces high concentrations of calcium in the blood, while PTH (parathyroid hormone) and vitamin D do the opposite.

A group of researchers at Cambridge University have found many reasons for suggesting that vitamin D has a hormonelike action. First, it is similar chemically to steroid hormones, and second, like hormones, it acts on the nucleus rather than on other parts of a cell. American researchers meanwhile have found that interference with the operation transcribing DNA (the nucleic acid in the cell that contains the inherited message directing the cell's functions) into messenger RNA (which executes the order in the message) can inhibit the action of vitamin D on calcium absorption. But much is still to be learned about this vitamin.

Our organism can synthesize vitamin D abundantly under sunshine, so, normally, we need not take supplementary doses of it. However, in cold regions or in urban environments where the ultraviolet radiation is filtered out of sunlight by glass windows, there can be a shortage, reflected in insufficient calcium levels. In fact, severe vitamin D deficiency can result in rickets. Since the 1800's when this was realized, vitamin D has been supplemented by cod liver oil or more recently by synthetic, capsulized doses and exposure to ultraviolet light.

An excess of vitamin D can be dangerous. This is a serious

problem because the vitamin is a common food additive. In the *Consumer's Dictionary of Food Additives,* Ruth Winter points out that pregnant women given too much of this vitamin can develop excessive calcium deposits, causing facial deformities and subnormal intelligence in their offspring. Nutritionists recommend about 400 units of this vitamin for pregnant women and children, but many women take as much as 3,000 units.

Vitamin E

Vitamin E is a fat-soluble vitamin, found in vegetable oils, green leafy vegetables, egg yolk, milk fat, nuts, and wheat germ. It is destroyed by deep-fat frying, rancidity, and ultraviolet radiation. The role of vitamin E is far from being completely understood, but it is almost certain that it is needed to protect cell membranes, for instance, to prevent red blood cells from breaking up. Malnourished infants with certain types of anemia have been successfully treated with vitamin E. It is also an antioxidant. Thus it may protect other substances, vitamin A, for instance, from oxidation in the intestine.

This vitamin may also have a role in the aging of cells, by protecting them against damage, notably damage caused by loose bits of molecules called free radicals, which we also discuss later. Dr. A. L. Tappel has described this hypothesis in *Nutrition Today* (1967):

For example, when radiant energy, which can penetrate throughout the body entering every cell, strikes a polyunsaturated lipid that is present as a nutrient, one of two things happens. If enough vitamin E is present, the radiation will have little effect. If, however, there is an intracellular deficiency of vitamin E, the energetic rays will strike a lipid molecule and knock loose a hydrogen atom. This would typically initiate the peroxidation of polyunsaturated lipid . . . (forming free radicals). The free radical flies about within the cell under terrific force and without any pattern to its movement until it strikes another molecule and causes all sorts of damage. Lipid peroxidation is, therefore, widely regarded as the mainspring in the aging process.

It has been proven that vitamin E is involved in the reproductive cycle of animals and that animals fed on a normal diet containing all vitamins have a breakdown in sexual activities if vitamin E is withdrawn. Vitamin E is undoubtedly beneficial to sexual functions (as are other vitamins), but it has not been proven that huge amounts of this vitamin, as some doctors recommend, have a particularly favorable effect in increasing sexual potency. In my experience, approximately 400 units a day is sufficient. Some of this requirement, of course, is available in our food. Wheat germ and rose hips are particularly good sources of vitamin E.

The Canadian physician, Dr. Evan V. Shute, has found that the daily intake of 400 I.U. Vitamin E can act as a preventive measure against cardio-vascular diseases. I always advise using the natural vitamin E rather than the synthetic, especially when high intake (mega-vitamins) are involved.

Vitamin K

This fat-soluble vitamin is necessary for the production of prothrombin, a substance needed for blood coagulation. It is widely distributed in nature (in green vegetables, in cabbage and cauliflower, and in liver), and you would practically have to starve to have a vitamin K shortage. It is also synthesized by intestinal bacteria. The only indication I can imagine for vitamin K prescription is to premature babies and in some cases to newborns whose intestines are still sterile.

Enzymes

This is another category of substances required by the organism. They are organic compounds, whose quantity in the body can be increased by cell activity. They act as catalysts and are often associated with vitamins. (Thiamin, a vitamin of the B complex, for example, is part of an enzyme system required for the digestion of carbohydrates). Enzymes are manufactured by your own body, but it is not known whether enzymes absorbed from other tissues (such as food you ingest) are useful in manufacturing them.

What is known is that if they are useful, you don't get them in cooked food. Enzymes stop working at very cold temperatures,

but they are not destroyed and are ready to work again when
the temperature returns to normal. But heating at 125 or 130F is
enough to destroy most of them. Since water boils at 212F and
meat roasts at around 300F, cooked food is no-enzyme food.
Some researchers believe that the absence of enzymes in cooked
food fed to zoo animals (or to cats if you remember Dr. Pottenger's experiment) leads to diseases similar to the diseases of
civilization.

Trace Elements

Like enzymes, trace elements are necessary to life. They must
be absorbed by the organism because it cannot produce them
itself. Many trace elements are known, and some are undoubtedly still unknown. Hardly a year goes by without a new trace
element being discovered as essential to man. Until 1957 only
seven trace elements were so recognized: iron, iodine, copper,
manganese, zinc, cobalt, and molybdenum. Since 1957,
selenium, chromium, tin, vanadium, fluorine, and silicon have
been added to the list.

They are not easy to identify, because only infinitesimal
amounts are required, measured in parts per million or parts per
billion, but their absence can provoke diseases whose origin is
often difficult to determine. A deficiency of selenium, for instance, can contribute to liver diseases or muscular troubles, but
so can many other deficiencies.

Until a few generations ago, nature provided us with our
daily requirements of trace minerals, but the plants from which
we receive them drew them from the natural nutrients in the
soil. Many of today's plants, grown in mineral-depleted soil and
fed with artificial fertilizers, do not have access to these trace
elements. This has been verified by tests: tomatoes grown with
artificial fertilizers, for instance, contain hundreds of times less
iron than naturally grown tomatoes. Overprocessed and artificial foods may have no trace minerals at all. This is certainly true
in the case of white bread, white rice, and sugar.

What can we do about this? We know that all of the trace
elements essential to good health have certainly not been

discovered, yet those we do know about are increasingly unavailable in our diet.

There is one obvious answer, and I am surprised that it is not widely recognized. It is sea water, the primeval element of all life, and it contains the trace elements. All the trace elements eroded from earth eventually find their way to the sea.

I do not mean you should drink sea water, although you could. Instead, boil a gallon or two of it down to a tenth of its volume, and after it cools, put it in the freezer. By the next day (or even in several hours) you will notice that crystals have formed at the bottom. This is pure sodium chloride (NaCl). Pour the liquid on top into a container, and use it for salting your food and cooking. Quite enough salt remains in it for flavor, and it also contains all known trace elements — and probably all the unknown ones. Discard the crystals.

This liquid concentrate you have decanted can be bottled and used instead of refined salt in cooking, salad dressings, soups, or anything that needs to be salted. By doing this, you can be assured of an adequate supply of trace elements. If you cannot do this as a regular practice, at least two or three times a year try to take a teaspoonful of the concentrate twice a day for two or three weeks.

Deficiencies of certain trace elements are associated with well-known clinical diseases. One example is goiter, resulting from a shortage of iodine, which the thyroid gland needs to synthesize its hormone, thyroxin (a regulator of energy metabolism). The thyroid gland becomes enlarged, and the condition is called "endemic goiter." This is well known in Switzerland, the Pacific Northwest and the Great Lakes regions, where the water supply and the locally grown vegetables lack iodine. If a pregnant woman's thyroid does not receive an adequate supply of iodine, her child may be affected with cretinism.

Iron is another important trace element (the body contains about as much as the weight of a penny). The principal function of iron is to become part of the hemoglobin, which, in the red blood cells, carries oxygen from the lungs to the tissues and carbon dioxide from the tissues to the lungs. Shortage of iron affects this transport, and the person feels tired and weak.

Again, an adequate supply is particularly important to the infant and the pregnant woman.

The average American diet provides 5 to 6 milligrams of iron per 1,000 calories, that is, about 12 milligrams a day, which may be insufficient. Chief sources of iron are organ meat (particularly the liver), egg yolk, leafy green vegetables, legumes, yellow fruit, whole grain, nuts, and raisins.

One way of increasing iron supply is to use iron pans, such as the old-fashioned cast-iron skillet, for cooking. Another way is to take an apple and drive a few iron nails into it. Leave the nails overnight, and eat the apple in the morning (removing the nails beforehand, of course). There is no danger of tetanus, unless you injure yourself with the rusty nail.

Calcium is another mineral of which there may be a shortage in the American diet, and it may be a major reason why many children have poor teeth. An infant's teeth formation starts during pregnancy, and unless the woman's nutrition has been exceptionally well balanced, an increased intake of calcium may be recommended (in the form of milk, which supplies calcium, phosphorus, vitamins A and B, as well as protein).

It is very likely that trace element deficiencies contribute to diseases such as arteriosclerosis, muscular dystrophy, cancer, cerebral arterial diseases, and some mental diseases, and this possibility is now the subject of research at several universities and medical centers.

11. *Plant Power*

Phytotherapy and aromatherapy are two ancient forms of medicinal therapy used by Egyptian, Greek and Roman physicians centuries ago. They are, of course, related. Phytotherapy is treatment with plants in general. Aromatherapy is treatment with essential oils, extracted mainly from plants, sometimes from animals (such as musk).

Both types of therapy are now undergoing a strong revival. Many scientists in Europe are exploring the power of these sometimes forgotten recipes. Professor Léon Binet, the late dean of the Faculty of Medicine of Paris, was one of the pioneers in this modern revival. Also in France, the medical faculties of Toulouse, Rennes, Montpellier, and Lyon now teach phytotherapy. In Italy, phytotherapy is taught at medical schools in Milan and Padua. There is a great emphasis on the medicinal use of plants in the Soviet Union. In Germany, several important pharmaceutical companies (Hoechst, Furth) prepare aromatic medicine. In the United States, phytotherapy is so far taught only at the University of Pennsylvania.

Research in aromatherapy has involved many attempts to analyze essential oils, which have mainly shown that these vary from year to year and from crop to crop. The oils are made of complex components, and some of them have been analyzed but never reconstructed in the laboratory. Some synthetic molecules or parts of molecules are used by the food industry to imitate natural flavors, but when it comes to therapeutic action, none of these synthetic molecules are effective.

A component that represents only one-millionth part of the essence may be the one that has the therapeutic effect, so it is much simpler to use essences provided by nature. Here, again, competition with nature is futile.

Applications and Aspects of Plant Therapy

Plant therapy can't do everything, but it can do some things very effectively and usually with fewer side effects than drugs. This is not to say that it shouldn't be approached with caution. Workers with vanilla plants are subject to vanillin poisoning, which manifests itself as headaches, gastrointestinal troubles, and oddly enough sometimes total (although not permanent) loss of eyebrows. Excess of saffron can overexcite the central nervous system and provoke severe convulsions. There are other such examples.

I wouldn't use aromatherapy for surgical anesthesia (although it has been done) nor phytotherapy for the treatment of a massive infection, although, in a sense, antibiotherapy is an extension of phytotherapy. The discovery of penicillin started with the observation that certain molds kill bacteria, and penicillin itself is but a plant extract. Aromatherapy can be very effective in the treatment of many frequent, minor, ill-defined ailments. These are usually treated symptomatically, that is, the symptoms are treated but not the cause, either because we don't know the cause or because we can't eliminate it even if we know it. Stress and carbon monoxide in the air we breathe are examples of such difficult-to-eliminate factors.

Plants perform no miracles. If they are therapeutic, it is because they contain therapeutic substances. Some of these we are beginning to know and analyze, but most of them have defied analysis and probably always will, because natural, live substances are infinitely more complex than man-made drugs.

Plants as antiseptics

Many plants or plant essences have an antiseptic activity. A few years ago, my friend Professor Griffon, whose wind-drier I have spoken of, tested aromatic essences as a means of bacteriologic purification of air. He mixed essences of pine, thyme, mint, lavender, rosemary, clove, and cinnamon. He then sprayed them by aerosol in a room after making a bacterial count in the room and placing some additional cultures in it. (Of course this is the idea behind commercial room deodorizers and purifiers, but they contain chemicals too. We are talking about natural plant essences *alone*.) Within half an hour, all the atmospheric bacteria had been killed, and some of the other cultures had been inhibited or destroyed. (A Staphylococcus culture was completely killed.) Another physician has tried the same in a hospital, where there were about 10,000 organisms per cubic meter. He simply placed a jar of essences in the room. In 20 minutes, 40 percent of the microorganisms were destroyed, in one hour, 80 percent, and in nine hours, nearly all.

You can make a powerful and fragrant natural room purifier yourself. Any combination of the essential oils of rosemary, lavender, and thyme will work. The combined oils should be dissolved into pure (ethyl) alcohol in a ratio of 4 to 10 percent oil/96 to 90 percent alcohol. Then, distilled water is added to the mixture to dilute it, pouring the water in gradually until the liquid begins to cloud. You can then put it in a bottle with a spray attachment for aerosol use. When the liquid is combined with baking soda, as described in Chapter 14, it is used as a skin tonic.

So aromatherapy is not a joke. The pharmaceutical industry knows this, and it is very fortunate for us that it is becoming more interested in the subject. It is beginning to use real plants or essences more frequently, rather than making drugs out of plants or making synthetic imitations that may not contain all the active ingredients. I am not crusading against the pharmaceutical industry, for which I do some research and which is providing us with increasingly powerful and specific drugs. The point is we must not overconsume these, because any overconsuming is harmful. Especially since nature has put an appropriate remedy at our disposal, why turn to the synthetic pill?

Plants for relaxation
The habituation to tranquilizing and sleeping drugs is a well-known phenomenon. I once had a patient who had been taking assorted sleeping pills for ten years. He couldn't sleep without them but, after getting used to a new pill, either couldn't fall asleep with it or woke up in the middle of the night. He was a British statesman, and I think he had tried all of the sleeping drugs available in England, constantly changing to the newer ones, and sometimes having to resort to pep pills to come fully awake.

Polite skepticism could be read on his face when I suggested that he try drinking an infusion made either with a mixture of orange flowers and leaves or with chamomile. I even gave him enough plants to make a few infusions, as I suspected he wouldn't go to the trouble of looking for the ingredients.

When I saw him again a fortnight later, he was off pills and had replaced his evening tea with a cup of the infusion I had suggested. Yet I discovered the extent of his skepticism at the beginning of the treatment when he told me that although he had promised me to try the infusion, he had not promised to abstain from the pills. So, on the first few evenings, he downed his pills with the infusion. The pills seemed to work better, and he decided really to give it a try. Fortunately the infusion worked with him — it doesn't with everybody, and sometimes the formula has to be altered. He had started by being so negative about "my herbs" that, had the first suggestion failed, I am sure he wouldn't have tried another.

Plants against the common cold

Another frequent abuse is the medicinal treatment of (or rather, the relief of symptoms of) head colds, benign bronchitis, or ill-defined, slight fever. The common cold, to begin with, cannot be cured. It is caused by a variety of viruses, too versatile and too numerous to lend themselves to the making of a vaccine. The only positive results have been obtained with interferon, a natural product secreted by a cell in defense against viral infection. But interferon is very difficult to produce in the laboratory, and so even this experimental treatment is very costly. However, this is our most widespread affliction. It is estimated that the average incidence is at least one cold per person per year. And we have seen hundreds of drugs on the market, presumably to fight it or its symptoms.

Symptoms of cold can be relieved by a highly effective but unfortunately not very tasty natural mixture: garlic and onion, boiled down to a thickish goo, to which honey and lemon juice are added. Two teaspoonfuls at night will give results that are likely to amaze. Breathing pine and thyme essences is also helpful. And to show you that I'm not always against synthetic products, take a lot of vitamin C.

Allergies and immunities

In the internal use of infusions or in the external use of plants, I have never seen a loss of efficacy with time, as there is with some drugs. Therefore, there is no need for progressively increasing dosages. At certain times, higher dosages may be needed, but it doesn't mean you can't return to lower ones afterward. You don't become immune to the effects. This isn't so with antibiotics, for example, which seem to create not only an individual but also an environmental need for increased dosages (which means simply that the organsims around become more resistant). We used to routinely administer 100,000 units of penicillin. Now the usual dosages are closer to one million, and some physicians have administered 50 or even 100 million units a day for several consecutive days.

As to allergies, you may be allergic to a plant just as you might be to anything else. Obviously, this must be taken into consideration when using plants for health.

Absorption through the skin

Aromatherapy is still little known in America, and there remains some skepticism about it, notably regarding the penetration of certain essential oils through the skin. It can be easily demonstrated that the skin is *not* impermeable to essences. I once made such a demonstration, at a conference at the *Maison de la Chimie* in Paris.

A German physician and his wife (who was, I think, a biologist) came up with the usual objection that essences cannot enter the organism through the skin. One of the displays at the meeting was an iron lung, the kind of respirator used by people who are paralyzed and cannot breathe on their own. I asked the doctor to get in it with his shirt off. I rubbed some essential oil of garlic on his chest — nowhere else. When the respirator was closed, there was no garlic smell whatever. Shortly therafter I asked his wife, who had stayed outside, to come in and kiss him. She was reluctant at first, but finally she agreed. When she did, she exclaimed that he had such a strong garlic breath he must have eaten garlic! He hadn't, of course, and she no longer doubted that the essential oil had indeed passed through the skin barrier into the organism.

Some Useful Plants

There is no purpose in listing all aromatherapeutic and phytotherapeutic indications — there are many books which deal exclusively with the subject. But I will give a few hints which I have found to be particularly useful.

But let me first define the term "essential oil." It is a volatile, odorant, oily liquid or wax, that is extracted from plants, either by vapor distillation, by squeezing the plant, or by collecting the liquid as it comes out of an incision made in the plant. Sometimes solvents are used to make essences, and sometimes the essence is extracted with the help of another substance from which it is later separated. The various essences and plants, roots, leaves, flowers, and so forth used in phytotherapy can be found in some pharmacies and health stores. Some people, including myself, find it more satisfactory to pick or grow their own whenever possible. The added advantage is that in the process, you breathe some fresh country air.

Sometimes the essence is ingested. Sometimes it is rubbed on or used as a bath mixture. Essences are usually taken by the drop (they are very powerful) on a piece of sugar. Infusions, on the other hand, use fresh or dried plant matter in liquids, such as teas.

Now, for a few examples.

Bergamot

Citrus bergamia is a kind of orange tree, and the essence bergamot is extracted from its fruit. It acts as an antispasmodic and gastric stimulant and is effective against digestive troubles. Bergamot essence is sometimes used in suntan lotions to accelerate tanning. Some people are allergic to it.

Cabbage

This vegetable, not eaten very often nowadays, used to be known as "the poor man's doctor." Its greatest shortcomings as a medicinal plant are that it is not expensive, does not come from exotic countries, does not have a highfalutin and complicated name, and is not labeled with a long and complex chemical formula. Some of the therapeutic elements in cabbage are beginning to be known, but far from all.

A researcher at the University of Texas, Dr. W. Shive, has extracted from cabbage a substance called glutamine, that can be effective in the treatment of gastric and duodenal ulcers. His findings have been confirmed by several studies, notably by Dr. Garnett Cheney, professor at the Stanford University Medical School.

If cabbage treatment is continued for a long time, there should be occasional interruptions of two or three days. Cabbage juice (some people don't like it straight) can be mixed with carrot juice. The only danger when too much cabbage is used at the expense of other food is that it can trigger goiter in persons susceptible to it. Excessive use of any single vegetable or fruit can have side effects. I remember reading in a medical journal about a woman who had become orange-colored after a prolonged diet based almost exclusively on carrots.

Cabbage can also by efficiently used as a gastric regulator. Cabbage juice, or else a mixture of raw and cooked cabbage, is a natural weapon against constipation.

The most outstanding quality of cabbage is its ability to accelerate healing and cicatrization, the formation of scar tissue. One who has never used it will be amazed to discover how cabbage speeds up the healing of a wound. This property is useful against ulcerations, hemorrhoids, eczema, and sometimes against acne.

This method of utilization is simple if somewhat lengthy. Either white or red cabbage can be used (and for such use, I definitely recommend organically grown cabbage, to avoid the potentially irritating action of chemical traces it might otherwise contain). The thickest, most colored leaves should be chosen.

If you have rectal problems, notably hemorrhoids, a cabbage leaf applied to the area in question several times a day can give more permanent, less traumatic, and less painful relief than surgery. For best results, the leaf should first be washed carefully, then all the filaments removed with a knife and the leaf squashed with a roller or a bottle. When the juice appears on the surface, the leaf can be applied. Several leaves can be packed one over the other and left there for twenty or thirty minutes — just sit on them while you read or watch television. At night, they can be held on by covering them with cellophane wrap and securing them with a bandage or a sufficiently tight pair of drawers or bathing trunks.

If you're allergic to cabbage (this is easily diagnosed from the unbearable itch), try the same method with leaves of a leek or else a slice of melon — less effective, but more easily prepared and very refreshing indeed.

Cabbage is also a revitalizing food, that should be taken now and then as part of a varied diet. I have mentioned that sauerkraut (the kind sold out of the barrel, not canned) is an excellent live food. But don't put it on your hemorrhoids.

Another hint: if you're out on a later night, and drink a bit too much, a good way to avoid a hangover is to have cabbage or leek boullion, or onion soup, before going to bed.

Chamomile

The flowers and seed of this flower are used either to obtain essence or, with the leaves, to make an infusion. Chamomile tea, made from the flowers, is an excellent, mild, natural tranquilizer that can be effective against insomnia. It also tends to reduce fever and is effective against the ill-defined aches and pains that accompany temperature elevations of colds and flu. Chamomile flowers can be bought in some drug and health stores.

To make an infusion, take a handful of chamomile flowers and boil them for ten minutes in a quart of water. Use less, of course, if the flowers are compressed. If you wish to make a single cup, use a teaspoonful. Do not forget to press the flowers before removing them from the cup.

Cherry stems

The stems should be dried in the sun, then boiled (about an ounce of dried stems to a pint of water). The resulting liquid is an excellent diuretic. It can be drunk hot or cold, sweetened with honey if you like. Cherries by themselves are diuretic and laxative, as described in Chapter 9.

Cinnamon

The essence, obtained by vapor distillation of leaves and bark, stimulates respiratory, cardiac, and circulatory functions. It is a good tonic when you are tired and can relieve menstrual troubles. An infusion can be made with half an ounce of bark (the kind you purchase in grocery stores) in a quart of water, or the essence can be taken after placing two or three drops on a piece of sugar. This can be repeated several times a day.

(Sometimes my patients wonder why I recommend the use of a sugar cube, and occasionally of synthetic vitamins and drugs, instead of natural products. As I have mentioned before, we should try to take advantage of everything nature has provided us with as well as whatever we have invented, to make our life a better life. A lump of sugar now and then won't make any difference, but the consumption of 100 pounds of sugar a year will. As it happens, cinnamon essence has a rather pungent flavor and a convenient way to take it is on a piece of sugar. Of course, you can also dilute it in honey or in a glass of milk.)

Lavender

This important aromatherapeutic plant grows in great abundance in the south of France, where the annual harvest can reach 300,000 pounds. Essential oils, extracted by vapor distillation, and flowers are used.

Lavender is antispasmodic, analgesic, and has tranquilizing properties. It increases gastric secretions and intestinal motility. Used externally, it is an antiseptic and accelerates the healing process.

One heaping teaspoonful of lavender flowers dropped into a cup of boiling water is used to make an infusion. The flowers should be left in the water for three minutes. This beverage can be taken three times a day, between meals.

Eczema can frequently be relieved by a lavender-based ointment. A handful of lavender flowers are mixed into a pint of olive oil, kept warm in a double boiler for two hours, and left overnight to macerate. On the following day, the mixture is filtered through a cloth, and the liquid used as an ointment.

A lavender milk can be mixed in a bath to achieve a sedative effect. Taken at bedtime, such baths can be very effective in the treatment of insomnia. (Sometimes these are found commercially prepared.)

The bactericidal properties of lavender essences have been experimented with and found effective against a number of pathogenic microorganisms, including the typhoid bacillus, diphtheria and tuberculosis bacilli, the pneumococcus, and hemolytic streptococci.

For beauty care, lavender essence is mixed with thyme and rosemary essences to make "Queen Margaret's Water," named after Queen Margaret of Hungary, who is said to have invented the recipe (which you will find in Chapter 14), having been a beauty adept throughout her life. It can be used for massages and skin aspersions to help keep the skin smooth and retard the appearance of wrinkles.

Lemon

This common fruit contains several vitamins of the B complex, as well as significant quantities of vitamins A and C. It acts as a cardiac and nerve tonic, has diuretic action, and is antianemic.

The essence is contained in pockets of the skin. Some 3,000 lemons are required to produce a quart of essence. The pulp of the fruit contains chiefly citric acid. When you twist a lemon peel, you can see tiny sprays coming out. When you do this over a dry martini, you can see the essence in the form of tiny oily droplets on the surface of the drink. (Martinis are not recommended as a means of ingesting substantial amounts of lemon essence.) Remember also that the surfaces of many commercially available fruits are tainted by pesticides. So if you use the skin of a lemon to make essence, try to buy organically grown lemons. These are now available in some stores. In France, where lemon and orange peelings are often used to make a kind of wine, even street markets have stalls with higher-priced citrus on which, sometimes, no diphenyl has been used.

Lemonade is one of the best drinks when you are feverish. Against overweight, take a lemon, slice it, add two flowers of chamomile, and pour a cup of boiling water over them. Let the mixture macerate overnight and drink it in the morning, before breakfast.

Linden

An infusion of *linden* (or lime) tree flowers has only one known pharmacologic action, that of a light antispasmodic, but it is also an effective sedative, not conducive to habituation. It was frequently used in the Serbian mountains by laborers tired after a long day's work, after childbirth, or during convalescence.

Onion

It has been known since antiquity for its tonic, anti-infectious, and diuretic properties. Regular use is an important factor contributing to general health. Onions contain sugar, vitamins A, B, and C, sodium, potassium, phosphates and nitrates, iron, sulfur, silicium, phosphoric and acetic acids, oxidase, and other enzymes. Vitamins and enzymes are, of course, destroyed by cooking, so onions are best eaten raw, either plain or marinated for a few hours in olive oil and added to salads, appetizers, and already heated soups.

Rubbed on the skin, oil of onion helps relieve the pain of bee and wasp sting. (In the case of a bee sting, the stinger may remain in the skin — don't forget to remove it.)

Thyme

Used as an infusion of leaves and flowered tips, or essential oil extracted from these tips, thyme is a general stimulant, antispasmodic, and intestinal and pulmonary antiseptic. It also tends to increase blood pressure. It is one of the most effective remedies in treating the symptoms consecutive to a common cold or a flu, and it also provides relief in asthma.

An infusion requires one branch of thyme per cup. Boil it a few seconds and steep for 10 minutes, taking three or four cups a day between meals. If the essence is taken, three or four drops (on a small piece of sugar) can be taken three times a day. Thyme, of course, is a valued ingredient in gourmet cooking; one of the simplest uses is to place a branch under a steak or hamburger that is about to be barbecued. The fact of its being cooked does not make it less useful. Because of its antiseptic properties, thyme is also traditionally used for the preservation of food, notably meat.

Turpentines

By no means to be confused with the hardware or paint store product (any use of which could be dangerous), these are also aromatic substances, made with resins extracted from a variety of conifers. They have expectorant and antiseptic properties, particularly useful in bronchial infections. Turpentine or balsam essences for inhalations are available in many drug stores and pharmacies, and there are capsules and syrups made with turpentine essences. The related terpin, a bihydrate of turpentine, is used in cough syrups.

Ginseng

This plant deserves very particular mention because of its powerful, general revitalizing effects. Experiments that many researchers, myself included, have conducted in the past few years have demonstrated that it has a marked effect on physical and mental performance. Ginseng extracts, in the form of capsules and powders, are available in some European countries and in the United States (where a variety of the plant is grown but seldom used).

The Oriental variety is known as *Panax ginseng.* In Chinese, ginseng means "man-plant," a reference to the resemblance of the plant's two tuberous roots to human legs. The plant is about a foot tall, the leaves usually have five leaflets, and there is a bright red clustered fruit.

The valuable part is the root. Ginseng roots have been the only uninterrupted American export to China since the eighteenth century. The export has continued whether China was recognized or not.

The therapeutic properties of ginseng have been known to Chinese medicine since time immemorial, and the plant, not easily grown, is still in great demand. It has also been used in Tibet, Korea, Indochina, Japan, and India, under various presentations, such as teas, tinctures, wines, pills, and unguents, for the prevention of fatigue, headaches, impotence, amnesia, problems associated with aging, and other assorted illnesses. It sounds like a universal panacea, and such a reputation is likely to irritate the scientifically minded. It is not a panacea but an active therapeutic agent with an easily proven efficacy.

Records show that the Dutch introduced it to Europe in 1610, and the first scientific discussion about ginseng was held at a meeting of the Academy of Sciences in Paris in 1697. It was temporarily forgotten until 1710, when a French Jesuit priest,

Father Jartoux, was given some ginseng plants while in China. He described it in a letter published in Paris in 1713. A Jesuit missionary in Canada, Father Lafiteau, chanced to read the letter and began, with the help of Indians, to look for the plant in Canada. He discovered some near Montreal in 1716 and published a monograph about it.

Ginseng was known to be very much in demand in China, and its discovery in Canada precipitated a minor gold rush. Thousands of Indians and Canadians started digging it out, selling it (for 2 francs a pound), and the *Compagnie des Indes* soon monopolized the profitable trade. But the boom did not last long, as Canadian ginseng was picked out of season and when the plant was too young. The Chinese were not satisfied, and the flourishing export stopped.

The North American variety of ginseng is not the same variety as the Oriental one. Its botanical name is *Panax quinquefolium*, and it doesn't have all the properties of the Oriental ginseng. Nevertheless, the early settlers in New York also collected ginseng and sold it to local merchants who shipped it to China. Philadelphia was the principal export center, and some ginseng was sent to Europe in the hope that it could be cultivated there. It never worked out.

For many years, sale of ginseng was an important resource to the early American pioneers. The Moravian Mission (New Salem, Ohio) relied heavily on ginseng sales (at $3.00 a bushel) for support. Daniel Boone was engaged in the ginseng trade and dug for the root himself. In the winter of 1787–1788 he started up the Ohio River with a boat carrying some 15 tons of ginseng. The boat overturned, but Daniel Boone was off with another supply in the fall of 1788.

The plant was very difficult to grow, and the trade was limited to what could be picked. As the growth cycle is rather long (6 years before the root starts to fork into its distinctive shape), the supply rapidly dwindled, and very few people succeeded in cultivating it.

In recent years, modern science has honored ginseng with its attention, and the results seem promising indeed. Some of the first scientific research was done in Japan and the Soviet Union.

(The Soviet Union has since completely stopped exporting ginseng, keeping its harvest for military purposes. It was discovered that with the use of ginseng, the accuracy of fighter pilots was increased, as was the precision and speed of the ballistics calculations of artillery personnel.) South Korea is now systematically cultivating ginseng as a state agricultural monopoly and a source of foreign currency.

Experiments to measure and classify the properties of ginseng have been conducted on mice. In two groups of mice, identical in litter, age, and weight, one group received the ginseng, and the other did not. The mice were then thrown into separate tanks of warm water. They swam until exhausted, and were picked up just before they began to drown. Swimming time, of course, was measured.

For the first dunking, which took place one hour after ginseng administration, the ginseng-treated mice were able to swim on the average 25 percent longer than the control group.

After the rescue, each mouse was dried with a hairdryer and given a rest.

Two hours after the rescue, they were dunked again. The mice had had some time to recover, and the point was to see whether ginseng helped them to recover. Again, swimming time was measured. In the second trial, ginseng mice swam 59 percent longer than the other mice.

Another test consisted of having rats climb up a rope that moved downward at the speed of 6 or 7 yards a minute. To encourage the rats to climb, an electric current was applied to the floor, giving an unpleasant shock if a tail touched it. Ginseng kept rats climbing 33 percent longer than their untreated brothers.

In more recent reports, the Soviet researchers (led by Professor I. I. Brekhman, of the Academy of Sciences, Vladivostok) found that ginseng extracts increase the organism's resistance to stress, activate electric currents in the brain, and reduce the depressive effect of drugs such as barbiturates. It also protects against radiation and nitrogen-mustard gas.

Some of the most interesting experiments with ginseng were performed by the well-known geneticist/gerontologist M. A.

(Zhores) Medvedev (whose political opinions have recently caused him some difficulties). Medvedev tried to determine ginseng's influence on mental performance. This is a difficult test to make, as many subjective and environmental factors come into play, but Medvedev came upon the idea of using a test group of the same age (21 to 23 years), living under the same conditions, eating the same food, and having the same work and rest schedules. They were military radio operators, trained to transmit coded messages.

It is known that the transmission of coded texts is difficult because there is no sense of what is transmitted. Normally, operators work in shifts of no more than three minutes without a break because it has been found that longer stints cause them to make an increasing number of errors.

A first test was made to make sure that the 32 men selected for the test gave similar performances, and a second was carried out three days later.

All 32 subjects were given a small drink, flavored with cranberry extract. A few drops of ginseng extract in alcohol were added to half of the drinks. To the other half, a few drops of alcohol without extract were added. Neither the radio operators nor the men who were to follow their performance knew the test group from the control group.

Speed of transmission did not vary from one group to the other, but, after the first three minutes, the radio operators who had received the ginseng extract made, on the average, about half as many mistakes as the control group.

As I have said before, there is no elixir of youth, and ginseng isn't one either. But in the multitherapeutic approach — the shotgun fired in the right direction, and the target being hit more or less frequently — ginseng is certainly an important bit of ammunition. Other studies have shown that ginseng increases the desire to work and the pleasure of work, that it strengthens the voluntary motor system and increases stamina. It may not be the panacea it has been traditionally believed to be by the Oriental people, but it can improve appetite, sleep, and memory, and counteract vertigo, fatigue, and headaches.

A Bulgarian physician, Dr. V. D. Petkov, using ginseng in the treatment of nervous and mental disorders, has achieved a positive stimulating effect tending toward equilibrium, without any unfavorable side effects.

Needless to say, I've put some ginseng pellets in my own shotgun. In the wide spectrum of revitalization therapies, I use ginseng extract in association with the vitamins and trace elements that are most likely to be missing from a civilized regimen.

I have made numerous tests which confirm this plant's wide-spectrum ability to act positively on physical as well as mental processes without giving rise to the subjective sensations of excitement nor the side effects encountered with the use of amphetamines and caffein. The activity of ginseng is long-lasting, and there are no withdrawal symptoms of any kind when it is interrupted. Side effects and toxicity are apparently nil. None have ever been observed in human subjects, and in animals, experimental doses equivalent to the daily absorption of more than a pound of ginseng extract by a man of average weight have produced no ill effects.

Although ginseng can be found in the United States, to my knowledge the Food and Drug Administration has not been approached to undertake the required experiments to market the extract as a medicine that may be particularly useful in geriatrics. Moreover, a comparison between the American and the Oriental varieties has yet to be made, and culture methods standardized.

But it seems to me that there is a good lesson to be drawn from this recent rediscovery. It is a lesson in humility or, at least, justified modesty. How often we, the somewhat self-satisfied and superior creators and possessors of highly specialized and sophisticated scientific knowledge, look down with scorn at the traditional, empirical methods that have prevailed for hundreds of years.

Legend is history with poetry. Recent analysis has shown that the concentration of the various active factors that have so far been identified in ginseng is highest during the sixth year of growth — precisely the time when ginseng, the man-plant, develops the two tubercle roots that have the appearance of human legs, and the time when it is traditionally considered to be ready for use.

It is not so unusual that knowledge becomes legend and legend becomes knowledge again. In archaeology, this has been amply demonstrated by the discoveries made on the basis of the *Bible* and the *Iliad* and the *Odyssey*. Ginseng is a tiny but actual example of this in medicine, and it may be interesting for you to watch in the near future as ginseng is rediscovered. In fact, in September 1974, I was invited to lecture at an international symposium on ginseng, where I presented a paper on its clinical use. I was amazed to discover how much progress had already been made by the Koreans and Japanese in the pharmacological studies of the root. Instead of a mysterious Oriental plant, in my opinion ginseng is a powerful weapon in the arsenal of medicine, and I foresee in the future a wide use of it.

In this chapter, I have tried to give you some idea of the power of plants. None of the preparations I have described are new. They have been developed throughout civilization, passed the test of generations, and should not be rejected simply because they are too simple and not the end product of our recent scientific knowledge. I have tested these and found them to be most effective and also the least bothersome to prepare.

I realize that some people tend to laugh when they are told to sit on a cabbage leaf. I don't mind if they laugh, as long as they do sit on it, even if only to disprove a method that comes from grandma instead of a sophisticated research center. But if you find that this or another one of the hints I have mentioned works, take a second look at some of the simple traditional methods that our civilization has rejected wholesale.

After all, I am not asking much. I would like you to become conscious, aware of the furnace inside you that keeps you going, not to reject something that is old only because it is old. And not to close yourself to the thought that there might be more in nature than in a million pills.

12. The Benefits of Sea Water

All life came from the sea. Tiny unicellular algae and bacteria were probably among the first living creatures that gradually evolved into more complex, multicellular organisms and, after tens of millions of years, into fish, the first vertebrates.

From the primeval sea that was at the origin of all life, some of these fish started conquering solid earth. Fossils of the primary era include fish with a double respiratory system, branchia and lungs. Fins, used for locomotion in mud and occasionally on more solid ground, turned into limbs. Amphibians were born. This slow evolution is mimicked during the transformation of the tadpole, a branchiated, fishlike creature living in water, into the amphibian adult frog, with lungs and legs.

Such are our modest, still little-known beginnings. But what *is* known is that we have taken with us and carry within ourselves part of the primeval sea.

Rediscoverers of Thalassotherapy

At the turn of the century, a French physician, René Quinton, made a study of the composition of different sea waters. He found that the concentration of fundamental elements contained in sea water varied from one sea to another, but that there was a consistent ratio between these different elements.

He compared sea water and body liquids of different animals, including man, and found that the proportions remained almost unchanged. The concentration is different, of course, being about four times higher in sea water than in plasma and higher in fish and amphibian — animals closer to the sea — than in man. But the basic elements, and their proportions with respect to each other, are about the same.

Dr. Quinton also showed that animals could survive with sea water in their circulation. He found that dogs, bled from one vein and receiving into another isotonic sea water (diluted with distilled water to the same concentrations as plasma) survived, and returned to normal, no matter how much sea water was introduced to replace plasma. There were no pathologic manifestations. Later, when Dr. Quinton practiced in Brittany and treated children suffering from infantile cholera (which is accompanied by dehydration), he used isotonic sea water injections. He observed that rehydration was more rapid than with an artificial saline (or Ringer) solution.

A few years later Quinton founded a therapeutic institute in Brittany based on the use of sea water. Thalassotherapy (from the Greek *thalasso*, the sea) was reborn.

The healing power of sea water was already known to Hippocrates. One of the first spas using sea water was built on the island of Cos, where Hippocrates is believed to have been born. Such spas existed throughout ancient history, to be forgotten during the medieval centuries. A British physician, Richard

Russell, reintroduced sea spas in the nineteenth century, and the first three decades of the century saw, throughout Europe, an explosion in thalassotherapeutic research accompanied by the creation of many spas.

Another French physician, Dr. Breton, established that hydrotherapy achieved better, more rapid results if sea water instead of plain water was used. His method took advantage of sea water's buoyancy to enable movements that are otherwise difficult. Dr. Breton's son continued his father's work in the 1930's, and the Germans became interested in his work when they destroyed his institute in 1940 while building the Atlantic Wall. After the war, thalassotherapy was widely used in Germany for the treatment of battle and bombing casualties (that have now been replaced by traffic casualties).

Thalassotherapy Today

Today, thalassotherapy is practiced in Europe by every country that has access to the sea. There are specific treatment regimens for several diseases, such as tuberculosis and arthritis, and general revitalization treatments aimed at building up body resistance to fatigue and premature aging. Many modern techniques have been developed and experimented with, and in some cases, immediate results can be obtained.

The bubbling sea water bath has a powerful action through a sort of massage of nerve endings in the skin and by its ionizing effect. Negative ions sprayed into the atmosphere have been shown to reduce blood pressure, to have a normalizing effect on the electroencephalogram, and a pain-reducing action. Near the sea, there is an abundance of these negative ions in the sea spray. Insomnia and anxiety are effectively relieved by sea water baths and massages and by the inhalation of spray, to which aromatic essences can be added.

The overall effect is undeniable, even though we still do not know the precise causal relationship between the many factors involved and the observed results. There is no doubt, of course, that the rest, the change of atmosphere, the distance from one's usual residence, the break in the routine contribute to the favorable results.

I chose the Bahamas as the site for a single institute to work with all known revitalization techniques because of the extraordinary quality of the unpolluted waters in that part of the Caribbean. Jacques Cousteau, the well-known French oceanographer who has studied life in practically all of the world's seas and oceans, has found that the waters of the Bahamas are among the cleanest, and that its reef life is the wealthiest in the world.

It is important that the water used for thalassotherapy be live, pure water. At Renaissance, we have studied the pattern of prevailing currents with dye markers, and we pump water through a 500-yard pipe that reaches out directly to an incoming current, so the water is constantly renewed. It is not idle fancy that live sea water has the best therapeutic effects. Sea water that has been boiled or bottled for a few days does not give the same results. This has been demonstrated in numerous experiments, notably those which involve transfusions to animals.

Thalassotherapy and Respiratory Ailments

Let me tell you about a particularly significant incident which occurred at Renaissance. An elderly gentleman came to me suffering from emphysema so severe that he could hardly take a few steps without puffing and stopping to catch his breath. He was given a series of thalassotherapy treatments, as well as treatments associating sea water with essential oils extracted from plants.

The oils are mixed with sea water and aerosol-sprayed continuously in a cubicle where the person sits. Breathing such a spray is almost equivalent to receiving an intravenous injection. The liquid is atomized in the very fine spray and, when inhaled, passes the cilia in the trachea and reaches the lungs. The substances in the spray are immediately absorbed into the blood and circulated through the body.

Two days after coming to Renaissance, the elderly man could, for the first time in years, breathe with relative ease. However, his condition was so severe that the effect lasted only for a few hours. After prolonged treatment, the improvement persisted for several weeks.

He returned to Nassau a few months later hoping again to achieve such a relatively long-lasting remission. But after the first treatment one of the nurses told me there was no improvement at all, and the patient could barely walk. Needless to say I was disappointed.

I then discovered that the water in the pressure tank used for the treatment had not been renewed overnight, because the pumping machinery was out of order. The water in the tank was clean and unused, but it was no longer fresh, live sea water.

As soon as the machinery was repaired, we gave him another treatment, and immediate improvement was observed. On the following day, the patient underwent another thalassotherapy and aromatherapy series, and there was further improvement. When the treatment was completed the effect, once more, was maintained for several weeks.

The improvement, however, never lasted for more than a few weeks after treatment, and it was difficult for the patient to keep returning to Nassau. Finally he moved from his home in the Midwest to Fort Lauderdale, where his condition improved, not spectacularly but more permanently, simply because he was near the sea and went regularly to the beach where he inhaled at least some sea spray.

I do not have enough experience with the treatment of emphysema to know how consistently relief can be achieved with thalassotherapy. But I and other physicians have observed that there is always at least some relief and often spectacular results in the case of respiratory disorders.

I think it is a pity that this method is not more widely used in a country such as the United States, which has one ocean to the east and another to the west and thousands of miles of seashore to the South. In Europe, the benefits of thalassotherapy have been so widely recognized that it is a policy of most governments and many private enterprises to encourage it. Treatment is frequently prescribed by physicians and usually covered by medical insurance plans or paid for by the social security organizations. In the Soviet Union, factory workers from the north have the opportunity to enjoy periodic rest and treatment cures in some 700 institutes by the sea, mostly in the Crimean region.

For a city dweller, spending holidays near the sea has an almost immediate beneficial effect. A slight wind can be sufficient to produce an aerosol effect. Sea spray is in the air, it is breathed in, it penetrates into the lungs and enters the blood circulation.

For us the sea is a vast reservoir of mineral water. It contains all the known chemical elements, and for many of these (because we come from the sea) the proportions are very close to those required by the human organism. We have seen that the surest way to get a sufficient supply of essential trace elements is to obtain them from the sea.

Live sea water also contains gases. The surfaces of the oceans and seas, seven times greater than earth surfaces, provide us with oxygen. For millions of years, the oceans have given us live food to eat and oxygen to breathe. Everything came from, and everything returned, sooner or later, not to ashes, but to the sea. This natural, harmonious cycle has only recently been disrupted by the dangerous gift of industrial civilization. Strange garbage now finds its way into the seas. It is no longer absorbed, no longer fertile, and it does not return to the cycle of life. It contains tars, lead, mercury, countless other industrial poisons that prevent oxygen diffusion and that destroy life-giving organisms.

Fortunately there still are, throughout the world, places where pure, live water is available. Live water regenerates with surprising speed, and this regenerative power should be taken advantage of. It amazes me, when I walk along the beautiful beaches of the Bahamas, to see people clustered, fifty yards away, around the swimming pool of the hotel, which contains not live sea water so readily accessible here and so rare elsewhere, but the cadaver of water, smelling of chlorine or of whatever else has been put into it to make sure it is dead.

Sea water has its own bactericidal properties. They were studied as early as 1936 by an American biologist, C. E. Zo Bell, and later by three French researchers, who confirmed in 1946 the antibiotic potency of sea water against pathologic organisms of gastrointestinal origin abundant in sewage waters.

Algae and Sea Mud

Algae and sea muds are among the most active elements of thalassotherapy. They are concentrations of the sea. Algae vary in size from the 1/1000-inch-long diatom to the 1,000-foot-long giant kelp. Many of them contain ionized trace elements, ready to use as biologic activators. They also contain amino acids (the building blocks of protein), vitamins, and, of course, an abundant supply of chlorophyll that permits them to assimilate solar energy and transform it into chemical energy for the construction of live, organic molecules, from water and carbon dioxide. Muds, collected along shorelines, are basically clay into which natural sea water elements have been absorbed.

Application of algae or sea mud directly to the skin has an excellent overall revitalizing effect, when combined with warm and circulated sea water baths, showers, high-pressure sea water therapy, oxygen and carbonic acid therapy, and underwater massage (applied with a jet that progressively depresses fatty tissues and muscles, activating cellular metabolism and achieving a powerful relaxing and tonifying effect).

Kelp seaweed is an excellent food additive, not for its nutritive value in terms of calories or proteins but for the concentration of sea elements it contains.

Women are particularly responsive to thalassotherapy. A woman's neuroendocrine system is more easily influenced by the tonic properties of a maritime climate. The pituitary, adrenal, thyroid, and parathyroid glands are activated, as is ovarian function. A complete diagnosis must be made with great care, as some forms of neuroglandular instabilities can be aggravated by the abrupt onset of the stimulating effect of sea water. But once the diagnosis is well established, thalassotherapy can do wonders in the treatment of migraine headaches, gastrointestinal troubles, and menstrual disorders. Dysmenorrhea, characterized by difficult, painful menstrual periods, can sometimes be completely overcome by thalassotherapy.

Thalassotherapy Against Aging

One of the preferential indications is the treatment of premature aging. Fatigue, characteristic of aging, can be relieved, muscular tonus increased, cellular metabolism improved. Tests show that thalassotherapy increases the contractile power of the heart without accelerating its rhythm, that it improves capillary resistance, increases basal metabolism, and slows down intracellular potassium loss. Sea water and algae give to the aging patient the benefit of their amino acids, vitamins, and essential trace elements. Pinpoint showers, directed at well-known reflex areas, achieve results that resemble some of the effects of acupuncture.

I consider thalassotherapy as an essential part of the multitherapeutic approach I have gradually come to adopt. Modern research into the potentialities of sea water has only started, and already dozens of precise, specific indications are known. Thalassotherapy cannot, any more than any other therapy, claim to reverse the order of things and make time go backward. But by reducing illness, pain, and organic malfunction, it contributes to our struggle for a normal, active, full life.

13. *Easy Exercise and Elimination*

Before leaving this discussion of what goes into our bodies, let me mention two small things you can do to help your body function. I say they are small things, activities easily integrated into your daily life, but their long-range effect can be great. They are part of the overall approach we can take to a longer, more vigorous life.

From one of your most important openings to another, you are a long and varied digestive tube. Nature has designed this as an efficient transit system along which merchandise moves in a smooth turnover, with an equally efficient garbage-disposal system at the end. But you must ensure that your digestive tube does not become a bulgy, loose, and inefficient container that invades the rest of your organism.

We lead lives during which we seldom use our abdominal muscles. Some of us may indulge in abdominal muscle-building exercises, but it isn't really fun to lie on the floor every day and do situps and legups. For most of us, these exercises are the exception rather than the rule.

This is a shame, since sufficient muscle buildup can be accomplished in a very short time and in a way that you'll hardly be aware of it.

I haven't invented these basic exercises, they're part of yoga training. Inhale as deeply as you can, and *then* pull in your stomach forcibly and hold your breath for a few seconds. At first this requires effort, but very rapidly it becomes easy. The point is to do it off and on five or six times a day, thus avoiding the drudgery of scheduled exercise, which one tends to give up.

I have learned that the best way to sustain this is to create a conditioned reflex. Many of the people I have treated, for instance, work in offices and therefore usually take an elevator. Exercise there on your way up or down — it is hardly noticeable, and it wastes absolutely no time. Once in the elevator, take a deep breath (sorry if the air is polluted, I can't help that). Then pull in your stomach, as hard as you can. At first, hold only for a few seconds, so as not to get a cramp. As you get better at it, keep the stomach tight for 10 to 15 seconds (usually less time than your elevator trip takes).

At first the exercise will be conscious, but it soon becomes a conditioned reflex. As the doors of an elevator close, you'll find yourself inhaling. Even four to six times a day is enough for your abdominal muscles to retain a good tonus.

Many people to whom I've given this advice admit it becomes compulsive. I remember one advertising salesman who told me that one day somebody in the elevator started a conversation with him. He missed his mini-yoga session, so when he reached his floor, he signalled a down elevator without thinking about it, and did his bit twice in the morning instead of once: going down, and going up again.

Another patient remembers taking an elevator en route to an appointment with me. Unconsciously he began his breathing reflex. When he relaxed, he felt a tap on his shoulder. He turned, and a stranger smiled at him and asked, "Have you been seeing Dr. Popov too?"

If you don't have your daily ration of elevator riding, find something else. The exercise can be done standing, sitting, or lying down. You can do it every time you start your car, for instance, or every time you go to the bathroom. The point is to create the reflex so you don't have to think about it any more.

My second hint is about elimination. One of the trappings of modern civilization is the toilet seat, which has drawbacks other than its not being a very hygienic device. Peasants in the field or natives in the bush have none of this; they squat. It is a comfortable position, it has the advantage of stretching key muscles and helping tighten others, and it uses the added impetus of thigh pressure against the abdomen to facilitate elimination. Squatting exercises the right muscles. (It is still used, not only in primitive countries, but in some highly civilized ones as well, as the position for childbirth.) In fact, many public facilities in Europe have not a seat, but two foot-shaped outlines to place your feet on with a hole underneath. In your own home it is worthwhile (and no more expensive) to install such a setup instead of the comfortable seat where many people tend to settle, newspaper in hand, to wait for something to happen rather than to make it happen. If you don't want this conversation piece in your home, there is another solution. Buy or build a small wooden stool and put it right in front of the toilet seat. When you sit, put your feet on it. You will find that your knees-up position is similar to that of squatting, and your lower abdomen is compressed by your upper thighs.

I tested this with more than a hundred people, giving them radiopaque barium and taking x-rays before and after defecation, with and without the stool. People who did not use the stool had, on the average, two ounces more feces remaining in the rectum than people who used the squatting position.

It is surprising how many chronic headaches can be cured using neither aspirin, embryotherapy, nor assorted headache pills, but rather this method of reducing the amount of feces remaining in the lower bowel, and hence lessening the absorption of toxins through the rectal membrane. (This absorption is very efficient indeed; medicine commonly given in pill form in North America is prescribed in many countries in suppository form.)

Undoubtedly, many more things can be said about what we put inside us. But this book is not exclusively about vitamins, nutrition, or exercise, nor do I recommend that each of these hints be followed to the letter. Some of them may help you but may not work for your neighbor, and you may find it worthwhile to try others, or to select for yourself those that give the best results. Above all, do not hesitate to discuss with your physician any problem, however minor, you may have. A hint that is insignificant to you may be revealing to your doctor.

14. Rejuvenating Your Skin and Hair

The state of your health influences your outside appearance, and your outside appearance, through ceaseless feedback in the mind-body unit, influences your state of health.

A clear skin, a good muscular tonus, the absence of excessive fat, and well-kept hair all contribute to prolonged youth and should be taken into consideration in the multitherapeutic approach to revitalization.

Plastic surgery can come into the picture, but unless it is the correction of a defect you were born with, it should be postponed until your natural self-repairing mechanism can no longer be stimulated for that particular purpose.

Your Skin

Skin care is extremely important, not only because the skin is your outer wrapper through which the world perceives your image. Your skin is not an inert envelope enclosing your body but a vital, dynamic system. It represents about one sixth of your body weight and contains one fourth of your blood supply. It is one of the most important avenues of elimination and the most important temperature regulator.

It is impermeable to water and gases. Certain ions (electrically charged atoms or groups of atoms) can cross the skin barrier, and viruses and very few bacteria can penetrate it. We have seen that the skin is also permeable to some complex plant and animal essences.

The outer surface is exposed to light, dryness or humidity, heat or cold, but its internal limits establish contact with the warm, dark, yet lively inner world of the organism. As long as an organism lives, skin doesn't wear out because it is made of several layers of constantly reproducing cells. The uppermost layer of the skin is a dead layer, made up of cells about to be rejected. Nevertheless, it remains supple and moist, because it is lubricated by small glands that secrete a variety of substances. Skin is also a receptor organ, keeping track of the changes in the outside world and transmitting to the inside information required for adaptation.

It reflects the functions of the body, and the best equipped laboratory cannot inform us about the organism's condition as rapidly as do outward signs on the skin, in the eyes, and on the mucous membranes of the body. Cleaning the skin from the outside is sometimes useless, because very few skin diseases are the result of exterior irritation. More often they are the external manifestations of the internal conditions of the body.

Skin does require care, if only to protect it from the constant assault of millions of particles of dirt and chemicals and to keep open some channels between the outside and the inside world. By improving your general condition, you improve your skin condition, and vice versa.

Yet, what happens? You — and particularly if you are a

woman — behave like a funny bird. You are willing to spend time, money, and effort to look for and buy the best available clothes, shoes, jewelry, and other outer trappings. But when it comes to skin, which is not only your wrapping but also an important part of your personality, you follow the advice of an advertising campaign or the opinion of a girl who was put behind a counter for the specific purpose of selling a line of products.

I have nothing against cosmetics; some are good, and some are even excellent. But what is very good for a million other people is not necessarily the best for you.

I can almost hear the question: "But what else can I do?"

Natural Skin Remedies

There are a few answers. One is to visit a specialized institute, but good ones are few, and some of them will be pushing their own products. You can also try all available products and find out, by trial and error, which are the best for you. This may take a long time. If you have serious skin problems, you should not hesitate to consult a dermatologist. But there are other, natural, and harmless methods that can prevent some of the damage caused to the skin. They are not too complicated. Unfortunately, most of them are very inexpensive, and this seems to be an important shortcoming.

I have been told, between the garlic and the onion, that I give stinking advice. I am afraid I shall continue, by recommending lanolin.

Lanolin

Everybody has heard of lanolin, but not many people know what it is. The word turns up on many labels, from shampoos to cleansing creams, but most lanolin used commercially is chemically treated. You should use crude lanolin. Not an artificial concoction of cosmetologists, it is the natural oil secreted by sheep, the substance that gives raw sheep wool its greasy feeling. When wool is washed, you end up with clean wool in one place and lanolin in another. Crude lanolin can be purchased in some hardware stores. It does not have a very pleasant odor, but it is not expensive. A full skin treatment might cost you as much as 25 cents.

Lanolin gives skin elasticity, which can prevent the development of some wrinkles. There are two kinds of wrinkles: character wrinkles and the others. Character wrinkles are gradually formed, from childhood on. They reflect your moods, your dispositions and they can be beautiful, if what they reflect is beautiful. If they are not, no medication can cure them. They should be left as a kind of warning about who you are.

The other wrinkles are not necessary, as they reflect nothing but the loss of skin elasticity. Their appearance can and should be delayed. In Victorian times, young ladies were advised not to move their faces too much and to avoid sunlight. This does not correspond to our modern way of life, so the best way to avoid these wrinkles is to use crude lanolin. A monthly application is sufficient. I know of no woman who would be unwilling to suffer the outrage of an offensive odor for one hour a month in return for keeping a beautiful skin.

The treatment should be started early, as a preventive measure before the wrinkles have appeared. Once a wrinkle is in the skin, it is too late. Lanolin should be applied following the direction of the prospective wrinkles and left there for an hour.

Spring water

The skin of the urban dweller is exposed not only to the particles in the atmosphere but also to hard and chlorinated water, containing many mineral salts. This contributes to skin dilation, which also reflects itself in loss of elasticity.

Our less civilized ancestors washed in morning dew. This is very pleasant, but not always possible to the city dweller. Distilled water or natural spring water, which is becoming more widely available, can be substituted to wipe away the outrages caused by tap water. Don't take a bath in distilled water; it is too costly. But use it at least on your face and neck. In Europe, natural spring or spa water in aerosol sprays is used for the same purpose, but this hasn't caught on in the United States yet. However, you could simply put the spring water in a bottle with a spray attachment.

Witch hazel

I would avoid most commercial astringents, although the tightening-up effect is desirable. There is one, however, that is excellent: witch hazel. Its chief shortcoming, again, is that it is a traditional and inexpensive preparation, and as a result, people tend not to believe in its efficacy.

Natural moisturizers

If your skin is too dry, moisturizing can be achieved, without fear of any unpleasant side effects, with some natural products. Squashed avocado, virgin olive oil, or honey, applied for 20 minutes and washed away with distilled or spring water, can give excellent results. A colleague of mine recommends squashed strawberries, smeared over the face; the problem is that they should be left on overnight, and this *can* be a problem.

Chamomile

If there is a slight inflammation of the skin, a chamomile infusion can be used to rinse the face.

Cucumbers

When there are no major skin problems, a natural and time-tested concoction made from cucumbers can be used for upkeep. If you have a juicer, make cucumber juice and apply it over the face with a cotton pad. Leave it on for 10 to 15 minutes, then remove it with distilled or spring water. If there is no juicer available, cut the cucumber into thin slices and apply these directly to your face.

Queen Margaret's Water

For general revitalization of the skin, I would recommend Queen Margaret's Water, which I have mentioned before. The Hungarian queen's long-lasting beauty (and amorous prowess) was attributed to massages based on lavender, rosemary, and thyme. Essential oils of those three plants can easily be purchased, and here is the recipe for the basic bath salt: five parts lavender oil, two parts rosemary oil, and one part thyme oil. If you mix together half-ounces as parts, you will be making about a four-month supply of the oil base. An ounce of the combination is mixed with one pound of baking soda, and shaken well for a month's supply of the salt. Twice a week, take a bath into which one generous spoonful of Queen Margaret's mixture has been added.

Firming the Breasts

Women frequently ask what can be done to improve the tonus of their breasts. Aside from silicone injections, which I would never, never recommend, and plastic surgery, a last resort measure, I know of only two remedies that can give good results. I have had them tried hundreds of times.

The first one is a home remedy: Take a large spoonful of the Queen's mixture and dilute it in a quart of water. With this, massage the muscles and tissues that support the breast: down the sternum, underneath and around the breast, up to the shoulder along the pectoral muscle. The massage should last between 10 and 12 minutes.

Next you'll have to do something that you might find less pleasant. Take a handkerchief, fill it with crushed ice, and repeat the same massage with it, in front of the mirror. Continue until the massaged area becomes red — this may take between a half-minute and five minutes. Because of glandular alterations during the monthly cycle, this massage should be done during the fertile period, between 12 and 19 days before the next scheduled menstruation.

The second way to increase the firmness of the breasts involves cell therapy, which we describe in Chapter 20. It involves the use of eight-or-nine-day-old live chick embryos. This requires either an incubator or the availability of incubated eggs. If this treatment is started early, when a woman is between 25 and 30 years old, and continued regularly, it can achieve remarkable results. It can be commenced and can show results any time up to menopause.

Three Types of Face Peeling

Another professional treatment that can achieve excellent revitalizing results is face peeling. One way of doing it can be dangerous. It has been known, in some cases, to trigger kidney disease and even death. This is chemical peeling, using resorcin (or resorcinol) obtained from various resins or made artificially. When it works, it can work well. The face may remain red and swollen for as long as a week, but the peeling is radical and effective for 12 to 18 months (after which you have to start all over again — with the same risk). Dermabrasion, the removal of the outer surface of the skin with a high-speed polishing disk, is another effective form of peeling, that requires the expert hand of a qualified physician.

A much gentler way, used in Europe and at Renaissance, resorts to natural proteolytic enzymes (enzymes that digest proteins). The enzymes are placed on the face with a liquid plastic mask that solidifies, and they are removed 35 to 40 minutes later. Dead elements of the skin, digested by the enzymes, come off, but live ones that resist enzymatic action remain unharmed. This method makes it possible to examine the dead skin under the microscope. Examination can reveal what it is lacking and this can be used diagnostically in determining follow-up treatment.

Biochemical Skin Remedies

In addition to natural remedies, some recent biochemical research has achieved interesting results and may well revolutionize certain aspects of skin care.

It is a fact that the normal skin has a certain acidity, expressed in terms of logarithmic concentration of hydrogen, known as pH, with values from 0 to 14. A pH of 7 represents neutrality, numbers above represent alkalinity, and numbers below acidity. Normal skin is acid, with a pH around 5.5. Acidity provides a protection against some ions and is a condition of health. Decreased acidity usually reflects metabolic disorders that lead to pathologic skin conditions.

Lipoaminoacids

A French biochemist, Jean Morelle, demonstrated a few years ago that acidity in the skin does not come from ordinary amino acids (the components of protein) but from fatty (or lipid) fractions known as lipoaminoacids.

Lipoaminoacids are synthesized by both animals and plants. They have a high natural acidifying potential and can penetrate the skin, crossing the epidermal (outer) and dermal (inner) layers rapidly, to establish a biochemical equilibrium. These lipoaminoacids, which have been synthesized by French researchers, have been shown to increase the resistance of skin to various aggressive agents, to stimulate the skin's cellular and metabolic activity, and to have an antiinflammatory action.

One of the first practical applications of lipoaminoacids was the preparation of a very effective antidiaper-rash cream, and more recently these substances have been incorporated in the formulation of hygienic and cosmetic preparations.

Morelle found that lipoaminoacids, like antibiotics, either can be very specific or can display generalized activity when applied to the skin or scalp: protection against alkalinity, defense against microorganisms, and antiseborrheic action, among others. They also appear to act on nail and hair growth (but not on baldness). Their potential seems promising indeed, and this is a good thing, for there isn't much to boast about in the field of skin care, which seems to have been forgotten in the stampede of medical and technical progress.

Nails

Both hair and nails are outgrowths of the epidermis and are important parts of your covering. Nails are made chiefly of keratin, fibrous proteins that form the basis of horny epidermal tissues. Nails contain calcium, and defective nails can be a sign of calcium shortage or defective calcium metabolism, which you should check with your doctor. In my experience with cases such as this, I have found that a simple way to treat this is to absorb the natural calcium components that exist in eggshells.

Choose an egg, preferably laid by a healthy country chicken (it will have a much thicker shell than any laid by the egglaying machines employed in egg plants.) Wash the egg and place it in a small wineglass, not much larger than the egg. Squeeze enough lemon juice into the glass to cover the egg. Leave it during the day at room temperature, and place it in the refrigerator for the night. The lemon juice attacks the shell, and in the morning you'll find the shell is thin and soft. Carefully remove the egg with a spoon, without breaking it. The remaining liquid is lemon juice and calcium that can be directly assimilated by the organism. Make a lemonade with it (using honey rather than sugar) and drink it. Repeat the treatment every day for two weeks. In most cases, the telltale white streaks disappear, and the nails become harder.

Hair

Hair is also an important factor in your appearance and your well-being. It can reflect your general state of health, but, even more important, your hair has psychologic consequences that have been recognized ever since Samson met Delilah.

The problem of hair is entirely different for men than for women. Man's endocrine system can predispose toward baldness, partial or complete, which is very rare in women. Women's concern may be to keep hair healthy and pleasing in appearance, while man's is to keep it, period.

Some men have a lot of hair, some start losing it in their 30's, some lose part of it, others become totally bald. In some countries hair is associated with vigor and manliness, while in others, a shiny bald head is a sign of virility.

Hair loss

Of course many men are concerned about losing hair. In our civilization, loss of hair is associated with aging, and, at a time when a man starts losing the appearance of youth, it seems to accelerate aging.

It is no consolation that the best way to make sure to have a lot of hair is to choose your parents. The tendency to baldness is a hereditary one, and sometimes there is nothing you can do about it, except to give up or buy a hairpiece. But sometimes you *can* do something about keeping your hair.

The question of hair is, by and large, little known to medical science. Hair, like eyelashes, or beard, is of no direct importance when it comes to man's health, although it does have psychologic importance and not only reflects other conditions but, via the mind, can create new ones.

Keratin, the material hair and nails are basically made of, is lifeless epidermal tissue, a kind of byproduct of life.

Yet, we do know a few things about hair. I have mentioned before that hair is fundamentally an inherited, genetic characteristic, but this genetic characteristic must manifest itself in some way. It must, because of hereditary predispositions and living conditions, general health, hygiene, and specific traumatism directed against hair, manifest itself in some way that becomes the direct cause of hair loss. And although medicine is incapable of altering the genetic predisposition, sometimes it can act upon the direct cause of hair loss.

Acne is an example. In acne, infection is present, provoked by microorganisms, but it is also dependent on the individual's general condition and susceptibility to it, notably on hormonal and nutritional factors. There is, so far, no specific treatment against it, and acne vaccines, although a few have been tried, are not effective. But there are several ways of relieving acne, hence, as widespread acne can provoke hair loss, there are several ways of preventing this hair loss, although no single way is uniformly effective with all patients. Acne is one disease, but 100 people suffering from acne can have 20 entirely different manifestations of it.

Shampoos

A normal scalp is slightly acid. Soap is alkaline. Where acid and alkali meet the reaction can be violent. So the first thing, then, is not to wash hair with soap. A majority of commercial shampoos are harmful, too, because they contain detergents, exactly the same detergents that are used to wash laundry or dishes. Detergents dry up the sebaceous glands in the scalp. Being constantly dried up, the glands tend to secrete more and more sebum, and the result is seborrhea. Sometimes it becomes a vicious circle — the more hair appears to be greasy, the more you wash it; the more you act on the sebaceous glands, the more they function; and the more hair gets greasy, the more you wash it, until there is less and less of it to wash. Even dry shampoos pose the same problem, being mostly just dry detergents.

Nowadays there are shampoos for different types of hair — dry, normal, oily, or dandruff-ridden hair. Most of these are better than the standard all-purpose shampoos, but before selecting one, you should know the condition of your own hair. If you live in a polluted city, or if you use hair creams to groom your hair, it can appear to be greasy, although actually it isn't.

I have found that for most types of hair, and particularly for children's hair, which is still undamaged, the best of shampoos (with apologies to manufacturers) is plain water — pure rain water if you can get hold of it, or distilled water. If you insist on using a shampoo, don't use it too often. If your hair is dusty or grimy from all the pollution it collects in a city, it isn't necessary to put it through the washing machine every day. Rinsing it with plain water whenever you're under the shower is usually sufficient.

If possible, do the last rinsing after a shampoo with rain water. This isn't always possible, and your hair must be subjected to whatever is used to purify city water. In that case, do the last rinse with water to which you've added a few drops of natural acid, lemon juice, for instance, or apple cider vinegar, so that it takes kindly to the natural acidity of your scalp.

Hair color

I needn't, I think, go into detail about the well-known harmfulness of most dyes and artificial rinses. They are mostly used by women anyway, and women, thanks to their endocrine system, stand much less of a chance than men of losing hair. There is one wonderful and tonifying natural lightening rinse: a chamomile infusion.

Unless you want your hair to become much lighter in color,

do not use it in a concentrated form. Make an infusion of one ounce of flowers added to a quart of warm water, with a teaspoonful of vinegar. The hair becomes softer, more supple, livelier, and acquires a lighter color. After four or five successive applications, you won't recognize it.

Hair problems and baldness treatments

If there is any kind of trouble — itching, dandruff, loss of hair, infection of the scalp — do not run to the barber, the cosmetics dealer, the hair specialist or hair clinic. Hair grows out of the scalp, scalp is skin, and a skin specialist is called a dermatologist. If your own physician can't advise you, the dermatologist should be the first person to deal with the problem and to determine the underlying cause, infection, localized anemia, hormonal imbalance, seborrhea, or whatever it may be.

Frequently these conditions can be treated successfully. Sometimes they can't, and if the dermatologist who knows about it tells you the case is hopeless and baldness approaches, then it isn't likely that the hair clinic will be of much help. You may just have inherited "pattern baldness" and should resign yourself to the intellectual look, unless you prefer a hairpiece or are willing to undergo surgical treatment with hair punches or hair patch transplants.

These two treatments have given results that are highly variable, but at least they are successful in some cases. This cannot be said of the many, many magic wonder treatments and ointments that have been, and continue to be, sold to willing but innocent victims of hair loss. I have done considerable research in this area, conducting my own experiments as well as following those of others, and including efforts with everything from bone marrow and incubated eggs to nicotinic acid. Satisfactory results simply cannot be guaranteed in all cases, and some of the treatments are very expensive and could even be harmful. I have known wealthy men who persisted with such treatments because it made them feel more secure, and factory workers who have paid nearly a month's salary for a month's treatment — a tragic waste.

The hair-punch transplant operation (devised by Dr. Norman Orentreich, whose work is described in Chapter 17) has been performed on thousands of people. Small tufts of scalp and hair are removed from the back of the head and the sides, where hair grows thicker, and are replanted on the front or the top to cover the bald spots. The patches must be small (one sixth of an inch in diameter), and 20 grafts may be required to cover a square inch of scalp. It takes a few months before esthetic results become apparent.

Surgically, it is a simple technique, but great care must be taken in selecting the places from which the hair punches are taken and to which they are transplanted. If you've decided to go ahead anyway, make sure to check the new hairline the surgeon has decided upon. A recent survey, published in the American *Archives of Otolaryngology,* indicates that some doctors are devising new hairlines seldom seen in nature. An example pictured in the article, was the creation of a dermotologist who conceived an inverted triangle coming to a sharp point low in the center of the forehead. Such a hairline can only be compared to something like the hairline of Bela Lugosi in one of his famous horror films. All things considered, you may prefer Yul Brynner.

Another surgical treatment proposed recently is the bilobe flap, using larger surfaces of scalp. It is too early at this writing to judge the value of this method.

From the top of your head to the ends of your toes, your skin and hair are the signs you give yourself and the outside world of what goes on inside you. As I have said, skin problems are indicators of deeper health problems, and these bellwether signs should not be ignored. By the same token, your outer appearance can affect the way you feel inside — a beautiful supple skin, shiny and lustrous hair, smooth hands ending in graceful, well-kept nails can enhance your feeling of youth and well-being.

But as an inhabitant of this civilized planet, your outer shell is constantly attacked by harsh and polluted elements. A daily routine must be established *before* problems develop. I have tried to give you an idea of some measures that can be taken to prevent aging signs and some curative measures to be tried when things go wrong. The rest is up to you — but don't hesitate to enlist the help of Mother Nature.

15. Teaching Yourself to Relax

One of my patients was an immensely powerful European industralist who, at age 38, had inherited the factories owned by his father and, with them, the burden of carrying on. He lacked his father's long experience and authority, but he plunged in wholeheartedly, sparing neither his time nor his energy. Less than two years later, when I met him in my office for the first time, he was a nervous wreck, exhausted, and looking 10 years older than he was.

He took a 10-day treatment that included cell therapy, and was in much better shape when he left. Based on his condition, age, and so on, the follow-up indicated he would not receive another treatment for three years, an interval pattern which could be sustained for the rest of his life. (The length of time any cell therapy treatment can reasonably be expected to last depends on individual factors, which vary greatly from patient to patient, but also on age: as a rule, the earlier the treatment is started, the less frequently it should be repeated.)

He called me again one year later. He told me how much he had benefited from the first treatment but also how he had suffered from the stresses and overwork that came with his new professional role. He felt he had the business well in hand, but needed a boost to tide him over a few more months until everything ran smoothly.

I advised against his taking cell therapy again, but he was dead set on it, and I knew he would go to another physician if I refused. Because I knew his particular problems, as well as what treatments I had given him so far, I agreed to his request for help. He assured me his difficulties were only temporary. I gave him another treatment, including cells, and saw that positive results were achieved. But I warned him that, come hell or high water, I would not give him another full revitalization treatment sooner than three years from then. He was sure none would be required.

A year after that, we met in the street, and he invited me to spend the weekend in his country home. It was a beautiful castle in the forest, and the weekend was extremely pleasant, except that, throughout our various conversations, I sensed he was exceedingly nervous and tense. It was spring and the weather was fine, but he had the air-conditioning on, wore warm clothing, and tended to stay indoors near the fireplace. The phone hardly stopped ringing; factory managers or business associates called for advice or instructions. He kept a pad and pencil ready to take notes and jot down figures. Weekend activities for him could not have been very different from his day-to-day work.

Finally the truth came out. Yes, he *had* met me accidentally in the street, and of course he was delighted to have me as a guest and hoped that I would come again. But now that I was here, what he really wanted to discuss was another full treatment, to help him go through yet another difficult period. He almost begged me.

I felt sorry for him, but at the same time, I knew that a third treatment including cell injections in such a short time span would not be good for him in the long term. I refused. He said he would go to another physician (cell therapy is widely practiced in Germany). I told him to go ahead, but that I would not be party to something that would be harmful to him. We talked about it for more than an hour, and he accepted my position. He remained silent for a while. I remember his pensive face, his handsome features behind a mask of unhealthy skin, and the nervous twitch at the side of his mouth. Finally he turned to me again, and his face was a plea for hope.

"What *can* I do?" he asked. "You see the position I am in, the responsibility, the problems that I have to face, the constant demands, and what this is doing to me. Isn't there anything?"

I asked him whether he would be willing to attempt a really radical treatment. His face lit up: of course he would.

I told him to wait a few minutes, and I walked out of the living room. I suppose he thought I had gone up to my room to fetch some vials of experimental and potentially dangerous drugs, but I only went out to see the gardener.

When I returned, I held a brick in one hand, and a huge pair of garden shears in the other. "This is your medicine," I told him, and explained that if he continued to drive himself as he had for the past three years, neither revitalization nor any other treatment would help. Indispensable people, I told him, are usually found in cemeteries, and if he didn't learn to delegate his power, trust others, and occasionally forget every detail of his complex business, there was no hope. At worst, I said, he might make a bit less profit or have to relinquish complete control of the reins, but so what? Was struggling for success really worth his driving himself to premature aging, ill health, and death?

I felt I had gotten through to him, and that the time had come for him to make a decision. I handed him the shears and the brick. "This," I said, "is to cut your telephone wire. And this, to throw at the window before taking a fresh, deep breath."

He hesitated, then smiled. There was a boyish twinkle in his eye as he took the shears and made them snap in the air before bending down and vigorously snipping the long black wire. By the time he picked up the brick, he was smiling broadly. In a clatter of broken glass, the brick sailed joyously out the window.

He stood up straight, proud of himself, laughed, went to the window, and took a deep breath. He looked different already. We went out for a walk, and by the time we returned, he was an entirely different man — younger, gay, pink in the cheeks. His making the decision, and the somewhat dramatic execution of it, had had a much greater effect than cells or drugs or any therapy addressing itself to the body would have. The point was to get at the body through the mind — and the feedback effect was instant.

A few weeks later I received a card from him. He had gone abroad for a holiday and was "having a ball." The business, he added, was doing fine, as far as he knew.

That was the first and also the last time I've used shears and a brick for therapeutic purposes, but many less spectacular though similar examples could be given.

Relaxation and Stress

That little story only illustrates that men and women working under continued stress often forget how to relax. The ability to relax is essential, not only for your health and well-being, but also to help you solve the very problem or problems that make you tense.

Napoleon was known for his ability to detach himself from a crisis, however serious. Even in the thick of a crucial battle, at Austerlitz, for instance, he was able to sleep for a few minutes at a time, as if to recharge his batteries. Churchill did the same.

During World War II, in 1944, I was sent to see Churchill, who wanted a first-hand appraisal of the situation in the Balkans. I arrived at the Admiralty at about three o'clock in the afternoon, and was told that the Prime Minister was *sleeping!* With Churchill, I learned the ritual did not vary much: he undressed, put on pajamas, and went to bed, unwinding completely in fifteen minutes of sleep.

I once talked about this need for complete relaxation, particularly at a time of crisis, with the late President Truman. He used a similar technique, but more discreetly, announcing that he "was retiring to study state documents." In fact, he said, he wanted to be left alone to relax or sleep for a short time.

Relaxation and Your Biologic Clock

This need for total relaxation is not limited to man. Over-exerted animals are known to fall asleep, from one second to the next. Horses, cows, and other four-legged animals can even do it standing up.

Biologic clocks are built into every living organism. They represent the response of our organism following millions of years of adaptation to the prevailing rhythms of nature: the circadian (daily cycle) of darkness and light, the weekly and monthly lunar cycles, the annual solar cycle. We are geared to these cycles, and any departure is a trauma to which we have to adapt.

After crossing the Atlantic in a few hours from one time zone to another, we are six or seven hours ahead (or behind, depending on the direction of our flight) of our internal clock. It takes time to adapt, at least a few days. Some functions take more time to adapt than others. At first, we adapt our sleep and wakeful hours, then, more gradually, our glandular secretions also fall in step. But during the first day after such a flight, we are not quite ourselves; we may be irritable, fatigued, and moody. I have often thought it was bad practice for statesmen to fly across wide time zones on the day preceding an important international conference or meeting. When the meeting starts, they are not yet entirely themselves. When such flights are frequent, they can result in prolonged instability. This is evidenced by the profound disturbances in the menstrual cycles of airline hostesses.

Relaxation Training

The ability to relax doesn't come naturally to everybody, but even an unusually tense person can learn it. And he is the one who will most benefit from it. Usually this learning must be gradual. Few people are able to will relaxation without training.

First, you must calm down. This can be done in several ways: thinking of pleasant events, of people you like, or imagining yourself in a pleasant situation. Sometimes, simply counting to 10 is a good start. While not exactly a new technique, it works.

I remember another one of my patients, a businessman, who complained that he couldn't help blowing up during board meetings when he disagreed with his staff or thought one of them had done something stupid.

"Just stop and slowly count to 10," I suggested.

"In the middle of a meeting, just stop? Why, it would look funny," he objected. I told him that if he could afford to blow up, he could also afford to stop and count to ten. "You don't have to do it aloud, you know."

I saw him a few weeks later. He complained that he couldn't blow up any more, and he found it frustrating.

"You don't have to count to 10 *every* time you feel like blowing up," I suggested. "It's not a bad thing to blow up now and then."

He looked at me as if I had given him the secret to a great discovery, and smiled. I imagine he was looking forward to blowing up again, at least at the next meeting.

The best way to start relaxation training is, in my opinion, by lying down, or sitting in a very comfortable armchair. After a while, it is sufficient to *imagine* yourself in a comfortable armchair.

Then think of pleasant things. Remember a race you won when you were a child, or a game you enjoyed, or any one of your most rewarding experiences. Or else, daydream of the future, positive daydreaming, that brings about a kind of nostalgia for the future, rather than for the past. You can create in your mind a favorable image of yourself. It isn't necessary to imagine yourself as Napoleon or Greta Garbo. Imagine a realistic situation, but a positive one.

It has been demonstrated that a state of relaxation cannot exist in the presence of negative emotions. Measuring brain waves with the help of electrodes shows that as soon as a negative thought is given precedence, the subject snaps out of the relaxed state.

A final bit of advice: don't relax while driving a car. Once you know how to relax, you may be able to do it, even behind the wheel. But do relax before a long drive, and if you are fatigued, stop on the way for a few minutes and give yourself the gift of a few minutes' relaxation. Actors know the trick. You seldom see them chatting with admirers during intermission. They are charging up for the next act.

Relaxing mind and body

The mind-body feedback is a strong one. In the mind-body unit, relaxation must be total, or else there is none. Either relaxation can be triggered in the mind, or it can start with the body, in a classical fashion: Think of your right foot, it is motionless, it becomes heavy; then of your left foot; and so forth. It does not matter where you start or whether you start with the body or the mind. Do whatever is easiest for you. The two are so deeply interrelated that one will follow the other. Some people find it easier to trigger relaxation in the mind, others in the body. The same goes for tensing up: when you tense one part of the body, the rest follows, and the mind becomes alert. When you are mentally tensed up, the body becomes tensed up too.

I am reminded of a story, not entirely irrelevant, of a Serbian peasant who had managed to send his son to school. When the son returned, the proud father asked him to speak to him in Latin.

The young man was far from fluent and told his father: "Fine. I'll speak to you in Latin when you ask me to, but only if you won't think, at the same time, of the word 'hippopotamus.' "

Of course, whenever the father asked his son to speak Latin to him, the word hippopotamus came into his mind. The son had successfully created a reflex that saved him from revealing his ignorance.

There is much that we still ignore of the functioning of the mind and of the relationship between the mind and the body, but even without the electronic machinery now available for such study, the relationship is evident. It is sufficient to see a golfer think out his shot, a pianist unconsciously tapping a tune with his fingers, or the smile on a baby's face when he makes sucking motions in his sleep and, presumably, dreams of the bottle or of his mother's breast. The traditional "power of positive thinking" is not a vain saying.

A series of experiments has been carried out with three groups of students, all of them basketball players. For a certain period, one group underwent no training at all. The second group actively trained by throwing the ball into the basket. The students in the third group remained, during the same training periods, prone on their backs and simply *imagined* themselves throwing the ball into the basket.

At the end of the trial period, the actual average score of the first group remained unchanged. In the second group, there was a scoring improvement of 24 percent, and in the third group an increase of 20 percent.

Imagined positive experiences have about the same positive effects as real positive experiences. The subconscious makes no distinction between a true or an imagined event, between dream and reality.

Relaxation by enjoying beauty

Civilization may have brought about increased stress, but it has also placed at our disposal unprecedented means to meet this stress and to escape from it, at least for short periods. For a very moderate sum, you can have in your home the world's most famous orchestras, the most prestigious directors and performers. Why not teach your children, from the earliest age, to appreciate this gift, rather than to become addicted to television, which conditions them to situations of stress rather than relaxation.

I have, in this respect, two personal experiences that seem to me conclusive. At home, I have always tried to keep the background of what seemed to be good music. My children have been exposed to it from birth, and all have become, without any prompting, music lovers.

With one of them I've had the time to try another experiment.

I purchased a number of inexpensive, standard-size reproductions of famous works of art and half a dozen corresponding frames. Every few weeks or so, I simply took out the pictures from the frames and replaced them with others. We never talked about this, and I imagine that he just came to expect that the decoration in his room should change occasionally, for no particular reason.

One day I had to make a trip to Madrid and took along the boy, who was then 10 or 11 years old. On the way to my appointment, I left him at the Prado museum, told him to walk around, and to try to remember the pictures he liked best. When I picked him up two hours later, all of the paintings he described to me were among the best-known masterpieces at the Prado. Yet, he had never seen them: the reproductions I had placed in his room were from other museums. But seeing reproductions of other masterpieces had developed in him the ability to recognize (perhaps subconsciously) and appreciate the qualities that make a painting great. It developed, in other words, his taste for beauty, one of the strongest positive elements in our life.

16. Using Biofeedback

The last chapter gave examples of subconscious training or education. But, I have mentioned, training to control the mind-body relationship can become very conscious indeed. With devices that keep you informed of the pattern of your brain waves and of the responses of the so-called involuntary physiologic parameters, you can learn to control not only your brain waves but your heart rate or blood pressure.

The technique used to achieve this is called "biofeedback training," a very scientific term for the very simple process of teaching your mind to control certain "involuntary" functions.

A distinction should be made between biofeedback and forms of electrical stimulation of the brain, such as are used in the sleep machine or in the treatment of mental diseases. Biofeedback does not involve any outside stimulation of the brain at all. The electrodes are used only to record what happens, and the subject, on his own, conditions himself to influence his brain waves.

The electrical potential of the brain can be recorded in the form of waves that differ in terms of amplitude (wave height) and frequency (how many peaks or cycles per second — cps). There are four principal wave forms in man.

The beta wave, in frequencies above 13 cps, is produced during normal conscious activity.

The alpha wave, in the range between 8 and 12 cps, occurs at random intervals during normal consciousness. If alpha waves are emitted continuously, the person is in deep relaxation, for instance, about to go to sleep.

Theta waves, in a range between 4 and 7 cps, usually occur during sleep, when a person dreams. They can also occur during wakefulness, when visual imagery, or hallucinations, take place.

Delta waves, in the range between 1.5 and 6 cps, correspond to deep sleep.

Alpha waves often occur in bursts. Every time you close your eyes, you probably produce a burst of alpha waves. The alpha state is described as "nonthinking," "letting the mind wander," or "relaxing completely."

It takes a few half-hour sessions for an average person to learn to recognize unmistakably his alpha pattern and a few more to conjure up the alpha wave and the complete state of relaxation that goes with it.

A continuous alpha state is in itself pleasant, and it can be very helpful when it comes to facing stressful situations. Biofeedback training can help an insomniac to go to sleep, first by relaxing into the alpha state, then slipping below into the theta pattern.

When there isn't time to go to sleep, the alpha state can become a sleep substitute, even during the working day, at the coffee break or after lunch. Relaxation that accompanies the alpha state helps recharge your batteries, but it offers you the advantage, if you are alpha-trained, to be able to snap almost instantly into the relaxed pattern, which is similar, in its brain wave form, to meditative states after a long training in Zen or yoga.

The alpha state represents a quiet mind. It does not mean it is inactive. It can assimilate information and be creative. Studies are underway to confirm the observation that persons capable of extrasensory perception generate low alpha waves. The scientific community is beginning to take seriously some of the unexplained phenomena of the psychic realm and to try to understand the extraordinary control that some Eastern mystics can achieve over their minds and bodies.

Therapeutic Uses of Biofeedback

Biofeedback has an important potential in the field of health. Many laboratories have succeeded in training some people to alter, voluntarily, not only their brain waves, but their heart rate, blood pressure, skin temperature, and muscle tone. Biofeedback can be successfully used against migraine headaches, cardiac irregularity, and hypertension.

Of course, it is no panacea against disease. Biofeedback for the time being is a tool to help you control your mind (a rather satisfactory achievement) and, through this control, to add positive elements to the body-mind unit that we are.

Given the environment we live in, and the likelihood that this environment is not going to improve from one day to the next, the potential applications of this new research represent a hope — revealed only in the past few years — that we are about to burst out of the limitations of what can now be considered as classical scientific medicine.

What is within our reach today would have been considered science fiction yesterday. The interest shown, both by the medical profession and by the public, for this new area of research means that it is going to be pursued actively and that there will be an increasing demand for the benefits it can bring about.

And this is only right, for we must not settle for anything less than the best we can achieve.

It is worth mentioning some of the research, and some of the practical results that have been obtained in a few years in the United States, where biofeedback has been pioneered.

At the Menninger Foundation in Topeda, Kansas, Dr. Joseph D. Sargent, chief of internal medicine, and Dr. Elmer Green have found that subjects could increase and decrease blood flow in their hands (and, as a result, increase or decrease hand temperature). They noticed that one woman, who suffered from migraine headache, recovered from it when she succeeded in rapidly raising her hand temperature by a few degrees.

They repeated the experiment with other patients and found not only that nearly everybody was capable of learning to increase hand temperature but also that in about three quarters of migraine headache sufferers, the pain disappeared or was relieved as a result. This form of treatment is now being studied and put to use in several other medical centers.

At the San Francisco Medical Center of the University of California, Dr. Bernard Engel had found, several years ago, that biofeedback training enables people to slow down and speed up their heart rate. Later, at the National Institutes of Health Gerontology Center in Baltimore, he and other physicians found that this could be applied to relieve the symptoms of premature ventricular contraction and paroxysmal tachycardia (recurrent attacks of rapid beating of the heart with abrupt onset and termination).

At the Rockefeller Institute in New York, Dr. Neal Miller's team, after succeeding in teaching rats to raise and lower their blood pressure, tried it on people, with partial success, and Dr. Herbert Benson, at Harvard Medical School, showed that people with normal blood pressure, as well as hypertensive patients, could learn to control blood pressure. It isn't clear yet how long these favorable effects can persist, but even these results, a few years ago, would have sounded like science fiction.

Another approach to hypertension has been tried by Dr. William A. Love, Jr., of Nova University in Fort Lauderdale, Florida, who has trained hypertensive patients in deep muscle relaxation, achieving on the average an 11 percent decrease in blood pressure.

At the Casa Colina Hospital for Rehabilitation Medicine in Pomona, California, and at the New York University Medical Center, biofeedback has been used to retrain partially paralyzed patients to use some of their muscles. In New York, a first series of experiments showed considerable improvement in nine out of ten patients.

Asthma, too, can respond to this new technique. Dr. Robert Kinsman, of Denver's National Jewish Hospital and Research Center, is trying to have people with tendencies to asthma build up resistance to asthma-provoking situations, and Dr. Louis Vachon, of Boston University, has been able to achieve some encouraging results.

In Montreal, neurologist Fernand Poirier has done pioneering work in the treatment of epilepsy with biofeedback. He has found that not only can patients recognize the approach of the cerebral storm that will provoke a crisis, but they can also learn to control it. He has found — in what is the world's longest experience with this form of treatment — that within six months an epileptic can achieve such a self-cure, and he believes that improved techniques can shorten this time to two months.

The applications of biofeedback are so widespread that the Army and Navy have undertaken studies showing that almost every person is able to control his skin temperature after no more than three or four sessions with the biofeedback machine. Such voluntary handwarming protects against frostnip and is likely to reduce the severity of frostbite.

A medical doctor who would have spoken of such potential applications of biofeedback a few years ago would have promptly been labeled as a charlatan or a quack. Today, this action of the mind on the organism is a recognized fact, and so is the potential of biofeedback in the treatment of mental illnesses and neurologic diseases.

Psychic Research and Parapsychology

Psychic research in general is becoming increasingly important and, although still controversial, may open up entirely new methods of disease control. Today, some 200 American scientists are exploring its potential, in centers such as the Menninger Foundation, the Maimonides Medical Center in Brooklyn, the Stanford Research Institute in California, and the University of Virginia Medical School. Hoffman La Roche and other important drug companies are exploring the possibility of training the mind to control stress, and even the Bell Telephone Laboratories scientists have looked into such areas as telepathy. It is significant that the National Institute of Mental Health has granted Maimonides Medical Center funds for research on extrasensory perception, and that the National Aeronautics and Space Administration has financed a program of research on extrasensory perception at the Stanford Research Institute. The business community, also, has become interested, particularly since two researchers at the Newark College of Engineering, John Mihalasky and E. Douglas Dean, have shown in a long-lasting experiment (several years) that successful executives seem to have a sort of sixth sense — intuition, or whatever word one can use to describe an inexplicable ability to predict the future.

The general field of parapsychology is, of course, still the subject of unproven and extravagant claims of charlatans, but at the same time, science has come to realize that there is something about the power of the mind, or the spirit, that does not correspond to orthodox concepts of medicine, physiology, and even physics. The mind, whether through electrical or electromagnetic fields it emits or through some other force still not understood, seems to have the power to act on matter, and particularly on the organism that supports it. Doctors have long known that "the will to be well" or the "will to live" has a potent influence on a treatment, yet this has never been explained in terms of biochemistry or physiology. The time has come for science to show interest in those recognized but unexplained phenomena that may open up a new era of medicine.

Part IV:
The Science of
Revitalization

17. Man's Search for a Youth Factor

Just as stress, the key aging factor, has been aggravated by the shortcuts and pressures of modern technology, that same technology has brought us closer to a scientific knowledge of a youth factor. I say "scientific" because there is certainly nothing new about the search for this mysterious and elusive goal. The lore runs through history right up to the present day. The mere promise of it has always attracted followers to the newest claimant to the secret, until he is deposed by yet another huckster.

The essential theory is that there *is* a youth factor. That something somewhere in life exists that can be captured to prolong youth or, at the very least, life itself. That is why we study the Hunzakut of Kashmir, the Indians of Vilcabamba, the Abkhazians of the Caucasus. That is why centenarians are interviewed by newspapers. Man is forever in search of the answer to the inevitable question: how can I stay young?

Modern, scientific man has made — and continues to make — many attempts to find the youth factor. We can describe only a few. Indeed, an attempt to fully record all experimental efforts in this area would fill several books the size of this one. But the work of these precursors of our current knowledge help illustrate the principles underlying revitalization. Many of these experimenters happened on their discoveries accidentally. Others were proven wrong in later years but their research helped put others on the right track.

Alexis Carrel: A Giant of Revitalization Research

The first scientific experiment that pointed to the existence of a youth factor dates back 60 years. In 1912, Dr. Alexis Carrel, a French-born physician and surgeon and fellow at the Rockefeller Institute for Medical Research in New York, was awarded the Nobel Prize for his pioneering work in vessel suturing that opened the way to modern vascular surgery and transplantations. (As I mentioned earlier Carrel was a great influence on my life.)

Carrel had already started on a new avenue of research: the maintenance of living tissue outside the organism. He wrote in the *Journal of Experimental Medicine* that a strain of tissue taken from the heart of a chick embryo was still actively alive after 16 months of independent life. The culture medium was the plasma of a hen, to which were added the juices of eight-day-old embryos — in other words, incubated eggs. In this medium, the rate of growth of the 16-month-old tissue exceeded that of fresh tissue. If the embryo juices were not added, the tissue died.

Carrel's experiments indicated that the cells of animal organisms do not contain the causes of their own death, and that given the elements of vitality existing in younger tissues, they could become practically immortal. He called these life-giving elements "trephones," from the Greek *trepho*, to nourish.

Thirty years after Carrel placed the fragment of heart muscle in the nutrient medium, Dr. Albert H. Ebeling, Carrel's long-time associate, reported it was still alive. The mass of tissue was regularly trimmed, as it doubled in size every 48 hours. If it hadn't been trimmed, its volume in 30 years would have exceeded that of the entire solar system. The culture actually was maintained until 1946. Yet, the maximum life span of a chicken is only about 10 years.

Lately attempts have been made to discredit Carrel. However, without his pioneering work, many later researchers would never have succeeded, or even tried.

Other Evidence of a Youth Factor

We have also learned from other animals. Take a mouse, the scientific researcher's favorite. Remove a patch of skin, from the back or the thigh, for example. With a local anesthetic the operation is quite painless.

Transplant this patch of skin onto another mouse, a younger one, but one of the same strain. The patch takes nicely. It stays alive and functional, receiving its blood supply from the recipient animal.

When the recipient starts growing old, carefully remove the skin patch, and transplant it to a younger mouse, still from the same strain or family. The patch takes again.

It can thus be maintained alive and functional through several transplantations. It goes on living when the original donor is long dead from old age. The skin patch, of course, is not immortal. At some point it, too, dies.

Now take a rat, the scientific researcher's second favorite animal. First a young rat, and next to it, an older one. A not too complicated but delicate operation links the blood circulation of the two animals. Vein to vein and artery to artery, the sutures transform two separate blood circulations into a single one. Arterial blood is pumped by the heart of the young rat to the old rat. It irrigates its tissues, becomes venous blood, travels to the old rat's heart, and back to the young rat again. The connection, called parabiosis, can be made permanent.

What happens? The old rat survives well beyond his normal life span. The young rat's blood has a rejuvenating effect on the older animal.

This experiment was done in the 1930's by the late Dr. Clive McCay of Cornell University. More recently (in 1972) a study was carried out by Professor Frederic C. Ludwig, of the University of California, on several hundred rats. He also came to the conclusion that the blood of younger rats transmitted "something" to older rats that made them live longer, even longer than litter mates who were not subjected to the trauma of an operation.

A similar experiment was done by Dr. Dietrich Bodenstein, of the National Institutes of Health Gerontology Research Center in Baltimore. His work involved microsurgery, because his subjects were cockroaches. Young cockroaches have the capacity to regenerate lost limbs; old roaches lose this capacity; but when old cockroaches were linked up to young ones, they were again able to grow new limbs.

Of course, biochemists have tried to isolate and identify this hypothetical substance, either a youth factor in young blood or an aging factor in old blood. Nothing has been identified so far, although it was established with some certainty that this substance is not any of the known hormones.

In spite of these and other experiments, it is understandably difficult for the medical establishment to accept the notion of a youth factor or of trephones or whatever one wants to call this "something" in a young organism that can revitalize an old one. Of course, no formula is known, and that is a great obstacle to its recognition. The ultimate aim of many modern scientific researchers is first to find the formula, then synthesize the stuff, and then find out if the synthetic stuff works as well as the natural one. There's a hidden trap there.

Take two nuts, one out of a can, the other fresh from the tree or from a country market. Apply the latest techniques of chemical analysis, backed up by the most up-to-date equipment.

You'll come up with the same chemical formula for both nuts. But there is one great difference. Plant both nuts into good earth. The first one will rot; the second one will grow. One is alive, the other one is dead. Alas, there is no formula for the difference. *Ergo*, there is no difference? I find that this kind of argument strains the limits of my patience.

A Soviet biologist named Oparin has spent much of his life trying to synthesize life. He made fatty globules, coagulates, and emulsions; he saw things moving and coalescing, but no life was synthesized. Others have tried to reproduce in their laboratories the crushing pressures of earth during its formation, the hypothetical ooze of primeval times, the Biblical thunder and lightning. Frankenstein's heirs keep trying, but still no life.

But the simple extract of embryonic juice and something in the blood of young animals do have life. And, beyond any doubt, it can renew life forces. Only life can give life. This fact, in my opinion, is the point of departure of any method designed to renew any vital supply. It is the basis of revitalization.

In the 1930's, when I became interested in the search for a youth factor, Carrel's tissue cultures had already lived more than 20 years, despite the fact that embryonic cells placed in a culture do not normally survive beyond 50 cell divisions (this was demonstrated recently by cancerologist Leonard Hayflick of Stanford University).

I read all Carrel's published articles, probably most articles published about him, and even published a few analytical articles myself about this field of research. What fascinated me most was the possibility of prolonging the reproductive capacities of cells without interfering with the rhythm of life. This was not an unrealistic idea.

Carrel and others had managed to increase the number of cell divisions beyond the normal 50 by adding embryonic juices to the culture medium. There is clearly *something* in embryonic cells, or excreted by these cells, that revitalizes the culture and permits it to continue growing well beyond its normal life span. It has been argued that cells in such a revitalized culture are no longer normal, but a similar treatment can be carried out on a living organism, with a revitalizing effect that prolongs life beyond its normal span. This was demonstrated in the experiment mentioned earlier regarding the two rats who shared the same circulatory system in which the older animal, receiving young blood, had a prolonged life span.

The existence of these revitalizing factors in young, and particularly embryonic, tissue forms the basis of embryotherapy, the programmed administration of live chick embryos, one of the fundamental weapons in the multitherapeutic approach to revitalization. The principles and applications of embryotherapy are discussed in detail in Chapter 19.

Modern Cell Therapy and Its Precursors

Cell therapy, another important part of revitalization therapy, involves the treatment of sluggish, ailing, or worn out organs or organisms by administering live vigorous animal tissue or cells. However, like embryotherapy, it is still reserved to a privileged few. Many people have never heard of cell therapy, or, if they have, they have been told it is the questionable brainstorm of a Swiss doctor named Niehans who died, in spite of his claims of having achieved rejuvenation, at the age of 88.

In fact, the idea of cell therapy is not new. Although Niehans can be credited with developing some important techniques in the area, cell therapy was known in ancient civilizations. One of the oldest known medical documents, the *Ebers Papyrus* (circa 1550 BC), tells of the benefits that the use of animal or human organs can achieve and even describes preparations made with organs taken freshly from animals. Traditional Oriental medicine has also treated deficiencies with the administration of fresh tissue. In the third century AD, Chinese doctors prescribed human placenta as a fortifying agent. Today, placenta tissue is widely used in cell therapy.

Homer wrote that Achilles ate bone marrow taken from lions to give him strength and courage, and Aristotle as well as Pliny the Elder mention that wolf liver was used against liver disease, and boar's testicles against impotence.

Paracelsus, physician and physicist of the sixteenth century, wrote that "the heart heals the heart, the kidney heals the kidney; *similia similibus curantur* (like cures like)."

The notion that blood contains a kind of youth factor was given credence by the fifteenth century Pope Innocent VIII who had blood taken from young boys injected into his veins. At the time, blood groups were not known, and an immunologic reaction must have taken place, since the Pope died shortly after the treatment. It would have been interesting to know the results of the experiment had he received compatible blood.

To the modern physician, the idea of rejuvenation through blood transfusion may sound farfetched, but then, isn't he applying the same principles when he gives an injection of blood-circulating hormones, such as thyroid or pituitary growth hormone, which have been extracted from animal glands?

In more recent history, Scottish physician John Hunter showed experimentally in the 1770's that roosters' testicles implanted into the gizzards of capons restored the latter's sex urge. This was the first documented experiment involving the transfer of living cells. The same experiment was repeated about 100 years later by A.A. Berthold of Göttingen.

All of this was confirmed in the classic scientific manner in the experiments of French physiologist Claude Bernard, who introduced, in the latter half of the nineteenth century, the concept of "internal secretion." Every physician today accepts the existence of the internal (endocrine) secretions described in Bernard's revolutionary theory proposed only slightly over 100 years ago.

There followed, at the end of the nineteenth century and the beginning of the twentieth, a few other significant attempts at cell therapy, including the two below which we described in some detail in Chapter 6. Most attempts were abandoned as unsuccessful, but one was retained, because it could bring consistently favorable results.

In 1889, Charles-Edouard Brown-Sequard, member of the French Academy of Medicine, injected himself with dog testicle extract and reported assorted favorable effects. But it soon became evident that the effect of this injection transplant was either subjective or very short-lived.

The famous Russian doctor Serge Voronoff tried a different approach: he transplanted strips of testicles from young chimpanzees to the testicular membrane underneath the scrotum of his patients. Voronoff's implants were all eventually rejected by the host organism. There was only a transitory effect similar to a hormone injection.

Paul Niehans: Pioneer in Cell Therapy

By far the most successful attempts to achieve rejuvenation with cell transplants were those of Niehans. In the early 1920's, when Paul Niehans was a young surgeon in Switzerland very interested in the new science of endocrinology, he had tried transplanting animal glands to patients as a permanent hormonal treatment of some deficiencies. In most cases the attempts failed, or provided only temporary relief, because of the host-versus-graft reaction, which hadn't been identified at the time. But in some cases, Niehans transplants succeeded at least long enough to achieve some results. One important success involved the treatment of dwarfism with pituitary transplants.

It was in 1931 that Paul Niehans did his first cell injection. It was an accident that he tried and an accident, I think, that he succeeded. The history of medical progress is paved with such accidents.

Niehans' reputation as an endocrinologist was already established when one day he received an urgent call from a surgeon colleague, asking him for help in what seemed a hopeless case. In the course of an operation to remove a woman's goiter (a condition not infrequent in Switzerland), the surgeon had unwittingly also removed the patient's parathyroid glands. Located just behind the thyroid, these glands control the calcium level in the blood. The woman had had tetany convulsions for several hours and was considered in a terminal stage.

She was in a hospital in Lausanne, ten miles from Niehans' home in Vevey. Niehans got off the telephone and went directly to the farm nearby where he kept experimental animals, had a young steer killed, and extracted its parathyroid glands. He rushed to Lausanne with them, but when he arrived at the hospital, he realized it was probably too late for a transplant. In a last-ditch attempt to save the woman, he made what was to be the first modern cell injection. He quickly chopped the steer's parathyroid glands into tiny pieces, put them into a saline solution, and, with a very large needle, injected the soupy mixture into a chest muscle of the dying woman.

In doing this, Niehans hoped to achieve the equivalent results of a hormone injection that might immediately relieve the spasms of tetany, so that he could then undertake a long-term treatment. However, either the parathyroid glands of the woman had not been completely removed, and the boost given by the injection restarted their functioning, or (and I think this is highly unlikely) the injected gland particles took and remained active, at least temporarily, to continue secreting their hormones. At any rate the woman survived for some 30 more years.

In the years that followed, Dr. Niehans proceeded with the development of cell therapy, using, as a rule, not the glands and organs of mature animals but those of unborn fetuses. He had closely followed Carrel's work and favored fetal cells because they seemed to possess, as did the chicken embryo juices Carrel had used to keep his tissue cultures growing, some vital factor.

In his search for this vital factor, Niehans solved another problem. He succeeded in avoiding the major obstacle to cell therapy: the immunologic rejection, or even worse, the generalized, massive rejection syndrome that can be fatal. This immunologic reaction is well known today. It accounts for the immediate or eventual rejection of transplants between two adults, unless they are closely related and share the same antigenic capacities. It was long after Niehans pioneered cell therapy that British zoologist Peter Brian Medawar's research proved the immunologic competence of embryonic tissues develops only after birth. That is, although the injected cells do not survive, their lack of antibodies means they do not provoke allergic reaction of the host organism.

In the 1930's, Niehans continued to explore many potential revitalization techniques, so it was not until the 1940's that he had fully developed cell therapy as one of revitalization's major weapons against premature aging.

Still, many skeptics were reluctant to accept Niehans' theories and chose to ignore the impressive results of his experiments. A number of other researchers have followed up on Niehans' work or adapted some of his findings to their own experiments, and, gradually, cell therapy has been refined, its applications widened, and its acceptance increased. I will mention only a few of the successors to Niehans to give you an idea of some of the more significant advances that have been made in the field of cell therapy.

Georges Mathé and Bone Marrow Transplants

In 1957, five Yugoslav technicians received lethal doses of radiation in a nuclear reactor accident. Strong radiation slowly destroys the bone marrow cells that produce lymphocytes, the immunocompetent cells of the organism. From previous experience, it was known that man can survive only a few weeks without lymphocytes, but the Yugoslav physician who was treating the technicians remembered that some marrow replacement experiments were underway at the Curie Institute in Paris. The five patients were flown to France, and their treatment was taken over by a young French physician, Georges Mathé.

Mathé found a number of human volunteers to donate some of their marrow to the Yugoslav patients. The marrow was extracted from sternum bone and immediately injected into the bloodstream of each patient. Although these foreign cells were eventually rejected by the host organism, they persisted long enough to produce the lymphocytes the organism was lacking and gave the patients' own marrow cells time to regenerate. (This form of cell therapy, incidentally, received official congratulations from the American Medical Association, which had previously and continues to reject cell therapy *in toto*.)

Georges Mathé, who has since received a professorship and government funds to create an institute of cancerology and immunogenetics, has adapted this form of cell therapy to the treatment of another disease: leukemia. In acute lymphoblastic leukemia, the lymphocytes are the cancerous cells. They reproduce in an uncontrolled fashion and invade the circulation.

Since lymphocyte cells destroyed by radiation can be temporarily replaced with injections of bone marrow cells, Mathé argued that by giving large doses of radiation — normally lethal — to leukemia patients, he could destroy the cancerous cells and then replace them with donor cells. With this form of cell therapy, he was able to achieve the first long-lasting remissions in cases of acute lymphoblastic leukemia, up to four or five years. But the treatment was not a cure, since the patient's own cells gradually began taking over again, and these cells were still cancerous. Faced with this hopeless situation, Mathé tried to give further bone marrow cell injections, but these provoked generalized rejection syndromes that could be lethal to the patients. Since then, drug treatment and immunotherapy have advanced to achieve remissions of up to 10 years, and cell therapy in leukemia is now used only in cases that do not respond to any other treatment.

At any rate, Mathé's work confirmed once more the transitory value of cell therapy. Foreign cells, even embryonic ones not rejected in a violent reaction, cannot be permanent implants, but the organism does draw from these injected cells the substances it needs until the foreign cells are eventually destroyed and absorbed.

Bullough Discovers Chalones

Recently another discovery was made which answers a classical question that had been raised against Niehans-style cell therapy: "How can cells from sheep, or lamb, or other animals, be utilized by the human organism, which is a totally foreign and different organism?"

This was partly answered by the proven fact that certain hormones, such as insulin and pituitary hormones, are active when extracted from animals and can be used in man. It doesn't work with all glands, but it definitely does with some. But a recent finding, still not widely known by the scientific community, gives more striking evidence of complex and still unidentified substances which can be transplanted from one species to the other.

For several years a British researcher, Dr. William Sydney Bullough, has been trying to isolate the hypothetical factor that encourages cell multiplication, perhaps the same one Carrel called "trephones." Through his efforts, Dr. Bullough discovered an *aging* factor, a substance which, rather than stimulating cell growth, acts to inhibit it. He calls his discovery "chalones," from the Greek, taken from a nautical command to take down the sails on a boat — in order to slow its progress. The aspect of his findings significant to cell therapy is that of tissue specificity. That is, the chalones he extracted from pig skin were effective in inhibiting cell growth on mouse skin, calf skin, and human skin, though not on pig liver, pig pancreas, or pig lymphocytes. In other words, not species-specific, but tissue-specific.

It is not known yet whether the amount of chalone in aging organisms is greater than in young organisms. It is likely, because cell division in old organisms is slower than in young ones. This is speculation. But the existence of factors which are tissue-specific and species-nonspecific no longer is speculation. This is the basic tenet of cell therapy.

Paul Weiss

The amazing degree of information programming in dissociated cells has been confirmed by another series of remarkable experiments, performed in New York at the Rockefeller University by biologist Paul Weiss, who, like Professor Bullough, is not a cell therapist.

The experiment consisted of taking, separately, the cells from various organs (kidney, liver, and so on) of a one- to two-week-old chick, mincing them, and incubating them in enzymes that break up the cells. The result is a clump of cells, which are washed and filtered to remove any residual matter. These cells are then deposited on a chorioallantoic membrane (the skin of the egg underneath its shell) and left there.

One might expect that the cells would rot or at best keep redoubling as cells in a culture usually do. Instead, the cells gather, as if purposefully preprogrammed, to form complete organ tissues. Kidney cells form tiny tubules, cells from limbs form cartilage surrounded by muscle, and heart cells link to one another to form a tissue that contracts rhythmically. Furthermore, an Israeli physician, Dr. A. Moscona, has shown that even mixed tissues of the same organ taken from *different* species come together to form a structure resembling the organ. I mention these rather esoteric experiments because I find it particularly irritating that much of the medical establishment persists in its stubborn rejection of the value of cell therapy.

Norman Orentreich

Many doctors may ignore or reject the notion of a youth factor because these experiments are not generally known among medical practitioners, few of whom would have the opportunity to test such a hypothesis in any case.

One brilliant New York physician is trying to do just this and seems to be achieving some favorable results. He is Norman Orentreich, better known for having invented a treatment for baldness which consists of transplanting small hair punches from the more densely populated parts of the scalp to the bald ones.

Dr. Orentreich, who had read of Carrel's work, and proceeding on the assumption that there is a plasmatic aging factor that exists in increasing amounts in older organisms, first experimented with dogs. He removed a dog's plasma, cleaned it, and reintroduced it into the animal's circulation. One of his dogs, treated regularly for several years, appears to have aged more slowly and to have retained more of his vitality and sexual powers than untreated dogs. Dr. Orentreich has since applied this treatment to human patients and believes also to have achieved favorable results.

Of course, such results are difficult to prove.

If someone today believed he had discovered a factor or serum which, administered during youth, could prolong the human life span by 10 years, he or his descendants wouldn't have any results to report until the middle of the next century. One way of judging the results of revitalization therapy (the way I have relied on) is to give patients regular tests and checkups, following the evolution not only of their organic function but also of their mental performance, by studying memory, intelligence, quickness of mind and of reactions. The comparison of these periodical observations with observations made on people who follow no treatment can demonstrate a slowing down of the aging process.

The evidence strongly suggests that youth factors do exist, but so far these factors can be transmitted only from one organism to the other, since they haven't been isolated. This is what happens in the experiments with mice and rats, and this is what happens in embryotherapy or cell therapy, which rely not on the extraction of a factor but on the transmission to an aging organism of cells from a young one or an embryo.

British physician Alex Comfort, who is by now better-known as an author, is probably the world's most renowned specialist on aging problems and research. He believes that some agent that demonstrably reduces the rate of mature human aging is likely to be known within 15 years.

Without saying so, Comfort also seems to feel, as I do, that joy is an important factor in retarding age, although he concentrates on that of sex. His books, *The Joy of Sex* and *More Joy*, have been tremendously successful. Such acceptance could not have been envisioned even a few years ago.

18. What We Know Today about Youth and Age Factors

Whether the youth factor is simply the absence of an aging factor or the aging factor simply the absence of a youth factor, we still have much to learn about what makes us grow old. Certain facts have been established and theories proposed about the changes that take place in an aging organism, and therapeutic programs have been designed to counteract these changes. I have incorporated some of these programs into my multitherapeutic approach to revitalization. Others I have found to be of little use.

A summary of these theories and related therapies follow to give you an idea of what can be done and what, unfortunately, is often done to no avail.

Free radicals

These are bits of molecules that seek other substances to combine with. Alex Comfort has described a free radical as something like a convention delegate away from his wife: A highly reactive chemical agent that will combine with anything that is nearby. Oxidative reactions with free radicals, for instance, make butter turn rancid. These reactions are harmful, as they interfere with the functioning of other molecules in the organism. The cumulative effects of such reactions contribute to aging. It was found that antioxidant chemicals that prevent these reactions can increase the life span of mice by 25 to 50 percent.

As it happens, there is a natural antioxidant available in food: it is vitamin E. Vitamin E is found abundantly in wheat germ and rose hips, which form part of our multitherapeutic approach to the problems of aging.

Cross-linkage

This theory, advanced by noted chemist and gerontologist John Bjorksten more than 30 years ago, holds that the aging of an organism is caused by the progressive formation of bridges between molecules. These bridges are irreversible. Once they are formed by cross-linkage they cannot be broken by normal cellular reactions or by enzymes. Gradually the tissues become stiffer, less elastic.

Bjorksten has attributed senescence to the gradual, progressive cross-linkage of molecules essential to life processes, since linkage prevents the molecules from functioning normally. The cells become clogged up with useless masses of cross-linked molecules, and they get into the way of normal reactions. If cross-linkage affects molecules in the nucleus of a cell, it can hamper the functioning of the cells' command posts, the DNA and RNA molecules that transmit vital instructions. Cross-linkage is encouraged by the existence of free radicals. Both of these theories undoubtedly correspond to at least part of the aging phenomenon.

It is suspected that the accumulation of food by-products not utilized immediately after the food is consumed increase the amount of cross-linking agents in the body. This may explain why underfeeding animals often increases their life span — every molecule of food is promptly used up by the organism, and there remains no useless material to participate in cross-linkage — and why our own tendency to overeat is related to premature aging.

It is known that radiation and the carbon monoxide in tobacco also increase the level of cross-linking chemicals. Bjorksten has carried out experiments indicating that atherosclerosis may be the result of cross-linkage.

Although Bjorksten has suggested that enzymes could be introduced into the organism to break up cross-links, this has never been achieved. It seems that the best way to reduce cross-linkage is to avoid the excessive accumulation of food by-products in the organism and also to reduce as much as possible the amount of free radicals through the use of antioxidants.

Autoimmunity

It is known that the immunologic competence of an organism is very low at birth and probably nonexistent during part of fetal life. As I mentioned earlier, this knowledge has encouraged the use of fetal organs or cells in organ transplants and cell injections.

With age, the immunologic system loses part of its ability to distinguish between good cells and bad cells. It has been shown that the production of antibodies secreted to fight off invading cells decreases with age but that the level of autoantibodies that attack the organism's own cells increases.

Dr. Roy Walford, of the University of California in Los Angeles, has performed a series of experiments involving the linkage of the blood circulation systems of animals (parabiosis) but with results opposite from those that had been obtained by linking together a young and an old animal of the same strain. In those experiments, the older animal, receiving presumed youth factors from the younger one, had a prolonged life span. In Dr. Walford's experiment, hamsters of *different* strains were linked together, but the result was that both animals aged more quickly, because there was an immunologic incompetence between them. Parabiosis had simply stimulated the autoantibody reaction characteristic of an aging organism.

Cybernetic theory

Dr. Joseph W. Still attempted to transfer the science of cybernetics to the specific problem of aging. Cybernetics is defined by its creator, the late Norbert Wiener, as "the entire field of control and communication theory, whether in the machine or in the animal."

It is known that the nervous and endocrine (glandular) systems act together as a control center to coordinate the activities of the organism. There is direct communication and feedback between the two systems, and according to the cybernetic theory, the symptoms of aging are caused by the slowed transmission in the nerve cells which are concerned with maintaining the system's harmony.

This is certainly a part of senescence, but there are really no indications that it is the principal cause of aging symptoms. With age, one does lose nerve cells (which are not renewable), but one also loses a lot of other cells. It is more likely that DNA, the genetic material that spells out the complex program for cell activity and replication becomes, after a time, less accurate, like a frequently played phonograph record that has many nicks and scratches.

Genetic errors

The overplayed-record theory also makes a lot of sense when viewed in terms of genetics. Geneticists have been puzzled by what is known as "redundancy" — the fact that many copies (sometimes thousands) of certain genes seem to exist in the DNA molecule. This doesn't correspond to the general pattern of economy and precision in nature, unless this redundancy was built in for some purpose.

According to a recent hypothesis made by Soviet geneticist/gerontologist M. A. (Zhores) Medvedev the purpose of the redundant genes is to fill in the scratches and nicks that are made as the original genetic material is used up — by mutations, for instance, that can be provoked by even tiny doses of radiation.

Redundant genes act as spare parts for these defective pieces. During old age, there are not enough spare parts, and the system makes an increasing number of mistakes. This makes sense, but it gives no hint as to what could be done about it, except, perhaps, through a general revitalization of the organism.

Senescence and sex

There is an intriguing relationship between the two. Once an animal is no longer capable of reproducing he is, biologically speaking, useless to his species. Remember the salmon who undergoes accelerated aging after spawning. Many other animal species exhibit a relationship between the reproduction cycle and longevity.

Many doctors have tried to treat man's senescence by enhancing sexual functions. We have already mentioned Brown-Sequard and Voronoff who worked in this area. There was also Eugen Steinach who developed the vasectomy, described earlier, to stimulate hormonal secretion.

Nowadays both male and female sexual hormones have been synthesized, and hormone-replacement therapy is currently used for both men and women. I have noted my reservations about hormone injections, and find also that as a rule, even when the injections are justified, they are not integrated into a wide spectrum of revitalizing therapies. Sexual activity is important, perhaps even the most important reflection of a man's vitality, but it is not the only one. Just as there is not one cause nor one manifestation of aging, there is not one single therapy.

It is much more effective to act on all of the components of the body-mind unit to achieve a natural continuation of the sexual function. This is not difficult, because there is nothing built into man's organism that determines, at such or such age, that sexual function should stop. Sexual glands, like any other glands, can continue to function as long as the organism is alive. This does not mean, of course, that they are as active as during youth. All glandular secretions in man slow down to a certain extent, reflecting a slower, although still totally active, pace of life. It is important to reject as total fallacy the notion that sexual function becomes worn out through use — it is the opposite that is true.

In women, the problem is different, because she is the victim, during menopause, of a sudden shortage of estrogens. There is no such clearcut effect in men. Yet, although the problem is different, the same error is often made: estrogen should not be the only revitalization therapy. In fact, the multitherapeutic approach to revitalization can delay menopause by as much as 10 or 20 years — or sometimes even more. As long as this delaying action is effective, there is no need to administer estrogens. But once atrophy of the ovaries sets in, it is an irreversible process. Then, and only then, should estrogens be administered, and they should be administered at the first signs of menopause to avoid the irreversible effects of total estrogen shortage. It is true that menopause, like diabetes, is a deficiency disease. It can be treated by providing the missing hormones, but then, as with other diseases, it is better to prevent it before having to treat it.

I have found that cell therapy, as it was developed by Dr. Paul Niehans, can be particularly effective against this when associated with other revitalization techniques. Revitalization therapy, started early enough and followed by estrogen therapy, can really postpone menopause. During the reproductive age, a woman uses up only a few hundred of the egg cells that are stored, in embryonic form, in the ovaries and released monthly. The total supply of egg cells, however, is 300,000 or 400,000. If we were to achieve, one day, a spectacular increase in longevity, the age of motherhood could also be considerably prolonged, provided these egg cells were not, themselves, damaged by aging.

We will leave now the search for the youth factor and the perhaps futile search for the *one secret* of a long life. But we take with us the readings scientists have made of nature, the rediscoveries of ancient healing arts and natural medicines, and we add them to our ever-growing multitherapeutic approach to revitalization.

As I have mentioned before, and will mention again, there are many things we can do to put a stop to the process of premature aging. Some of these things are complex and highly specialized treatments which should be undertaken by a trained specialist after proper diagnosis only. Cell and embryotherapy, for instance, are not home remedies and certainly should not be attempted as such. They are serious medical interventions and, like all effective medical treatments, can have secondary effects that might be dangerous if not properly supervised.

On the other hand, there are a number of treatments, habits, and regimens which you can adapt to your own life. Everything from improving your diet with the addition of live foods, to reducing the stress content of your environment, maintaining proper weight and indulging in a rich and pleasurable sex life are all activities which you can safely and effectively administer yourself.

19. *Modern Organic Clinical Procedures for Revitalization I:* Embryotherapy

Embryotherapy is one of the most effective forms of revitalization. It is absolutely harmless, there are no unpleasant side effects, no counterindications (except an allergy to eggs), and most important of all, its efficacy has been demonstrated in countless experiments with animals and clinical trials with people.

As a young medical student working with Ranko, I was intrigued by my mentor's insistence that live elements were needed to sustain life. A few years later I met Dr. Axel Munthe, the Swedish physician best known for his book, *The Story of San Michele*, and stayed with him for two weeks in his home on the island of Capri. He too insisted on the need for live food, and I remember clambering with him over the rocks of Capri to look for *lupari*, a kind of small clam, which we ate on the spot.

But all of this was, one could say, a young man's fad. It made sense to me, but I had done no research or experimentation.

Projekt Jot

At the end of World War II, I was assigned to Krefeld, Germany, where I was to treat recently released Yugoslav prisoners of war. They were a sad-looking lot. They had lived for many months, sometimes years, in unbelievable conditions of discomfort, overcrowding, and malnutrition. Many of them were mere skin-covered skeletons, such as most people have seen only in photographs of Nazi concentration camp survivors or starved Biafran dissidents. I started a rehabilitation program with whatever means were available — at that time, food was less than abundant.

While in Krefeld I met a young German doctor who had been drafted into the army. We talked, as doctors do, and one day he happened to mention a wartime research project in Linz which had involved not only German but other European doctors as well. Its aim was to test Alexis Carrel's chick-embryo trephone theory on human patients. My early interest in Carrel's experiments was rekindled, and needless to say, I was intrigued.

I managed to requisition a car and drove to Linz to track down the project, called *Projekt Jot* (yolk).

Somebody told me it had been carried out in an old castle not far from the city, but when I got there, I found out the Russians had already requisitioned and sent to Russia not only all of the doctors and scientists involved but every document and bit of equipment. As to the chickens, they had been eaten. The only person who knew anything about *Jot* was an old *Putzfrau*, a cleaning woman the Russians hadn't bothered to export. She knew little, but enough to intrigue me even more. She told me that eggs were incubated for seven to nine days, whereupon they were eaten raw by the experimental subjects (including some of the scientists). She didn't know a single name, nor any of the results, but said she knew the people felt better after taking the eggs.

I was reminded again of Carrel who reported that his culture medium worked best when supplemented by chick embryo juices after eight or ten days' incubation of a fertilized egg.

I drove back to North Germany determined to continue *Projekt Jot.*

I had in my convalescing POW's the ideal captive population for the tests. There were no ethical problems whatever. I knew that swallowing a live embryo was harmless, and the results could be at worst nil or at best positive. Shortly, incubators were requisitioned, and arrangements were made with local farmers for a supply of fertilized eggs.

First I tried embryotherapy on myself. I certainly needed some form of revitalization, and the early results seemed encouraging, although I couldn't be sure how much the improvement in my condition was due to the more regular life I was leading and the better nutrition in general, and how much to eating the incubated eggs.

Then I tried some very simple experiments on animals. I gave old ferrets, who love raw eggs, some incubated ones. Within two weeks their furs had clearly become more brilliant, and their behavior more lively. It was hardly conclusive or scientific, but it was encouraging. By then my egg supply had increased, and I began some large-scale clinical tests.

The POW's arrived in groups, so whenever a new group came, I divided it in two, trying at least approximately to match the men for age, general condition, weight, hemoglobin count, and muscular strength. The groups varied in size, but the largest were 100 POW's each.

The trials were really double-blind. Each man was given one raw egg a day. I had them swallow the whole egg through a hole in the shell, which was no problem because it is a Serbian custom to eat raw eggs in this manner. There was no way to determine, either by looking or swallowing, which eggs were incubated. Neither I nor the orderly who distributed the eggs knew which were which. There was a woman in charge of marking eggs, and she had her own code but she didn't know which eggs were given to what group of prisoners.

A month after the treatment started, I compared results. All the prisoners, of course, were by then in much better health. But the improvement was greater, on the average, in those who had received the incubated eggs than in the others, based on the results of the three objective tests — weight, hemoglobin, and muscular strength — used for comparison.

Some of the patients being treated with embryotherapy asked me about improving their memories. In undernourished, stressed people, memory loss becomes endemic, but I had not thought of including memory tests in my study, assuming memory would gradually return in both treated and untreated soldiers. However, I now added some primitive memory tests. The men were told to read a few sentences and recite as much as they could remember, or to look at a list of numbers and then repeat them backward and forward. A number of such tests were followed up for several months, and the difference between treated and untreated POW's was striking. Memory was recovered, on the average, much more rapidly by the men who had received embryotherapy than by those who had taken nonincubated raw eggs.

However, there was one POW I remember particularly well: a colonel who had once been a chess champion. He had lost his ability to play during captivity, because he couldn't recall the moves or tactics used in previous games. When he heard he had been part of my experiment with incubated eggs, he came, bursting with enthusiasm, to tell me that this gobbling of eggs for 15 days had improved his game fantastically. Needless to say I was also enthusiastic, as I thought this an excellent example of the improvement that embryotherapy could achieve. But alas when I had the records checked just to be sure, I discovered that the chess-playing colonel was in a control group — he had been eating plain eggs rather than incubated ones. Of course this didn't alter the overall results that were based on statistics that included several hundred people.

Another effect of embryotherapy soon became obvious. Many of the men suffered from secondary impotence and were unable for some time to have an erection, whether by self-stimulation or in the presence of a woman. The men, of course, tried to fraternize (as the military euphemism has it) with local girls, and one day an orderly handling the records remarked that the men on the embryotherapy list fraternized much more successfully than the others.

I questioned the men about this, and the responses, checked against the records, revealed that embryotherapy did speed up the return of normal sexual function. Fraternization records were then kept and compared in several paired groups, and they indeed showed the balance of improvement weighed heavily in favor of embryotherapy.

My assignment in Northern Germany drew to a close, and I left for Eboli in Italy to rehabilitate other groups of POW's. Once there, I continued the experiments. The test groups were larger and well paired, and the results of the first experiments were completely confirmed.

But before I left Germany, I had learned, to my regret, an unfortunate lesson about experimental techniques in the hands of careless amateurs. The press had become interested in the work I was doing. Several reporters visited me and talked to prisoners, and embryotherapy's favorable results were played up with such sensationalism that a hasty, poorly controlled practice in embryotherapy sprang up, using what became known as "Trephone Eier" (eggs) and even "Popov Eier."

It was too soon, it was done too hastily, and it was a terrible botch-up. But it served as an object lesson and warning of the dangers inherent in even the best of therapies when practiced by the uninitiated.

Growing embryos is not simple. Not only must the eggs be fertilized, but also one must make sure that the embryo starts growing and doesn't die. In my experiments, the condition of the embryo was constantly and carefully checked, and unusable eggs were boiled and reused as chicken feed. But in many of the overnight Trephone Eier enterprises in Germany, such precautions were not taken, and there were many cases of food poisoning (never lethal, but *very* unpleasant) in people who had eaten dead fetuses.

Infection is the most severe potential danger of embryotherapy: egg embryos, it is well known, are among the best culture media for viruses, and many vaccines, from polio to rabies, are made with virus strains grown on embryonated eggs.

Principles and Techniques of Embryotherapy

Aside from giving positive, controllable results, embryotherapy is absolutely nontraumatic. I do not claim it is rejuvenating, but it is certainly revitalizing, and the thousands of observations I have made in Germany, Italy, France, and more recently at the Renaissance Center in the Bahamas have confirmed this beyond any doubt.

But embryotherapy is not a fountain of youth. There are many tiny small springs that meet to form rivulets, that converge into streams, that meet in the stream of life. We do not know the secret of longevity. Most likely there isn't *one*. But we are beginning to know many secrets of vitality, and whenever you have a glass of water to add to the spring, you add it. Embryotherapy is one such source of vitality, and even as a single therapeutic tool, it is a powerful one, acting on the organism in the vital fashion the chick's embryonic juices acted on Carrel's tissue cultures.

When I had finished my assignment at Eboli after the war, I moved to France where I continued my researches in embryotherapy. I worked in Paris, but I got a farm in the South of France where I hired a Yugoslav expatriate as caretaker and started raising black Bentham Leghorn chickens. Each batch of chickens was coded, and I had the eggs sent overnight to Paris via the railway system that brought daily flower deliveries to the capital.

Although I had no trouble persuading the Serbian POW's to suck the raw eggs out of their shells, this is not a common habit of city people. For my new patients at first I simply broke the shell and placed the contents in a glass. If the subject was particularly faint-hearted, I quickly mixed the contents with fruit juice in a blender. Then I realized that swallowing the white of the egg wasn't necessary (remember Projekt *Jot?*). This made it easier, and today at Renaissance the embryo, less than half-an-inch long, is simply given in a glass with some of the yolk. Most people swallow it without batting an eye. This is the method now most widely used in Europe, and the result appears to be the same as if the whole egg is taken.

I also determined that the incubated eggs need not be taken continuously. Regular one- to two-week treatments calling for daily ingestion of an embryo taken from the incubated egg give excellent results. These one- or two-week regimens can be repeated five or six times a year — every nine or ten weeks.

The standard objection to embryotherapy is that the embryo, precipitated into the stomach and mixed with the digestive bolus (the mass of chewed food), is simply taken apart by the digestive enzymes. This is true if the embryo is administered during digestion. But when it's taken on an empty stomach, there is plenty of time for trephones (or any other name you may choose for the growth factor) to reach the bloodstream through the lining of the digestive tract. It takes only seconds, for instance, for water drunk on an empty stomach to reach the bloodstream.

Biostimulins

I left Paris and went to the farm in the South of France to study the notes I had taken on patients following embryotherapy and to try to establish the conditions under which the best results had been obtained. This was not easy, because this time I had not had a captive clinical population nor a double-blind and controlled study from which to draw conclusions.

I noticed, however, that one batch of chickens, batch number 23, had given particularly constant results. Not uniformly better but, on the whole, much more stable and predictable. This was confirmed by a comparison of blood counts, memory tests, muscular tests.

I thought at first this might have to do with the age of the chickens. I had wondered earlier whether the age was of any importance and asked that some of the chickens be cooped in age groups. When I went to inspect batch 23, I was told that the chickens had suffered from coccidiosis, a common barnyard disease, and had been taken away. Coccidiosis is not transmissible to humans, but I wondered what it was that made these eggs, laid by sick chickens, more effective than others.

Then I remembered the work of Vladimir Filatov. While making retina transplants, he had discovered that suffering tissues produced the biostimulating substance that encouraged growth of surrounding tissues. I wondered whether the coccidiosis embryos weren't more effective exactly for the same reason: they suffered and, therefore, produced biostimulins. I also recalled my own tomato plant experiment, and the healthy crop produced by the row which had lost a quarter of its plants in the early stages.

To test this theory, I didn't consider inoculating some of the chickens with the causative agent of coccidiosis, but I did think of subjecting them — or the embryos — to stress. Any form of suffering, I thought, might achieve the result.

I tried quite a few things: noise, in the form of a loudly played phonograph record or radio, and ultrasound vibrations; I thought of reducing the eggs' oxygen supply or adding gases to the atmosphere they breathed; I even tried x-rays.

I was experimenting with some of these methods, and talked about it one day with Brigitte, a bright and charming young lady I knew who had become quite interested in my work and occasionally helped me with it. She listened carefully as I described my attempts, then shook her long hair and burst out laughing. "I think I have an answer", she said. And indeed, she had; it was as simple, and as effective, as Columbus' egg. (The story has it that when Columbus was challenged to make an egg stand upright, he took a hard-boiled egg, cracked one end, and stood the egg on the cracked part.)

Brigitte suggested that I stand the eggs up in the incubator, and turn them around now and then, forcing the embryo (who generally settles in the upright position, head up) to struggle against gravity.

Normally, an egg that has been laid stays in the horizontal position, either under the mother hen or in the incubator, until it hatches. When the hen sits on it, she moves it about slightly, so that the yolk does not stick to the inside of the shell, and a similar motion, controlled by a clock mechanism, is made in the incubator.

Brigitte's idea worked perfectly, and it was, I must admit, infinitely simpler than x-rays, ultrasound machines, or oxygen deprivation. We cut out small circles in the wooden shelves of the incubator and placed the eggs head up on these circles. The embryos slowly settled in position. On the next day, we turned the eggs over and, observing them against the light, could see the embryos, head down, struggling to turn around. Some embryos died in the process. Normally, out of 100 fertilized eggs, I ended up with 80 to 90 live nine-day embryos. When I turned the eggs upside down every day, I had only some 60 survivors. But they were the fittest and those who had, presumably, succeeded in producing enough biostimulins to survive.

I began to make some tests to see whether there was really a difference between the distressed embryos and those developed under normal conditions. I conducted my tests not on human subjects but on mice. The same general criteria were applied — weight gain, changes in blood formula, activity (for mice this was measured on a treadmill). Memory tests were replaced with maze tests. These experiments showed that the biostimulated incubated eggs gave better and more constant results than those that had been left in peace.

Brigitte and I were delighted with this finding. It was not the first time she had helped me with the solution to a problem, and it wasn't to be the last. She also had — to an extent few people do — the gift of joy. We had shared many fascinating hours, and found in each other constantly renewed sources of enthusiasm. (Nevertheless, I must admit that it took me nearly eight years to persuade her to become my wife.)

Embryotherapy Today

Embryotherapy is now used by many physicians in Europe, and there are chicken farmers who specialize in egg-embryo production. But it is not as simple as it may seem. The health of chickens and the possibility of infection must be very painstakingly controlled. Production must be geared to a very precise demand — if an egg is not used at just the right time, it must be thrown away. The shelf life is limited to a few hours. With biostimulated eggs, an average loss of at least 40 percent can be expected.

Sometimes extracts of the chick embryos are made and given as injections. Other embryos can be vacuum dried. In some cases, embryos of other animals are used. I still believe the simple method of taking the chick embryo orally is the safest and most effective.

In order to start incubating the eggs, you must also have the required number of fresh fertilized eggs at the right time, and fertilized eggs, too, cannot be kept for long. Finally, the viability of the embryo must be checked within minutes before it is administered. (Some attempts have been made at freeze-drying the embryos or keeping extracts in ampules, but I have personally never been satisfied with the results.)

In the United States, embryotherapy is not available, simply because neither the medical profession nor the public is aware of it. No large-scale experiments have been carried out, and only a few physicians have started embryotherapy for themselves and their families. There is, of course, not sufficient demand for commercial production and distribution of egg embryos. Even if there were, an embryo could cost from two to three dollars, somewhat more if it is biostimulated.

I want to remind you that embryotherapy is not a form of self-medication, since there is, in the production of incubated eggs, the potential risk of infection and also the risk of consuming a dead embryo, which will be at best useless and might upset your stomach.

There is no doubt that, sooner or later, embryotherapy will be available in many countries outside of Europe. It takes an amazingly long time for an idea — and particularly for a medical idea that does not fall within the established pattern — to cross a border. Perhaps the most striking example of this slow process is acupuncture. Used in China for thousands of years, acupuncture was introduced to Europe by a Jesuit missionary at the end of the eighteenth century, and developed (particularly in France where it is practiced only by medical doctors) in the late 1800's. Nonetheless, it took over a century and a half in the United States before it was considered as anything more than quackery, practiced (illegally) only by a few initiates who were not medical doctors.

Acupuncture is now studied in the most respected medical centers and practiced by an increasing number of physicians. We can only hope that in the near future, embryotherapy too will enjoy the wide acceptance it deserves.

20. Modern Organic Clinical Procedures for Revitalization II: Cell Therapy

Cell therapy is another important technique for revitalization. Its principles are similar to those of embryotherapy, its results equally convincing. All the same, cell therapy remains a controversial subject, and physicians in some countries reject it completely, just as they have rejected acupuncture, despite overwhelming evidence that it is an impressively successful *medical* technique.

More than a million people in the world have benefited from cell therapy. It is practiced all over the world, and in Germany alone, over 4,000 physicians use it either for revitalization or as an adjunct to other treatments. More than a thousand clinical reports and dozens of technical books have been published about it. Public knowledge of cell therapy, however, is scant — aside from the fact that such celebrities as Pope Pius XII, Charlie Chaplin, W. Somerset Maugham, Konrad Adenauer, and Winston Churchill have been treated with cell (or cellular) therapy.

Lyophilized (freeze-dried) cells are prepared in Germany under the control of Heidelberg University and the Ministry of Health. These cells are shipped in sealed ampules throughout the world. (Even to the United States, where their use is not authorized by the Food and Drug Administration.)

The Principles of Cell Therapy

As we explained in Chapter 17, the theory behind cell therapy is that embryonic cells contain vital elements that can reinforce the functioning of aging or deficient cells. The basic tenets of this theory have been proven to be valid in experiments such as those I have described — notably Carrel's experiments with tissue cultures — and in embryotherapy.

In fact, cell therapy as it is now practiced is really a highly specialized form of embryotherapy. In order to treat deficient or degenerated cells of specific organs, the cells of those same organs are extracted from animal embryos or in some cases from young animals, cut into tiny pieces, mixed in a saline solution, and injected into the muscular tissues of the patient.

The precise action that takes place is not known, and in that respect, cell therapy does not differ from a number of widely used and approved drugs.

In the United States and Canada, the medical establishment, by and large, does not recognize cell therapy, although the overwhelming majority of doctors who are outspoken against it have neither experimented with it nor studied the abundant scientific literature published on the subject. When I encounter this narrow attitude, I am tempted to quote famous physiologist Claude Bernard, who wrote that "experimental results should not be adapted to theory; rather theory should be adapted to experimental results."

I started using cell therapy in the early 1950's, when I directed the Centre Médical de Récherches et d'Applications Biologiques in Paris. Several French physicians were using cell therapy, but a number of questions about it remained in my mind. There is a French saying that if you want something done, it's better to ask the Good Lord rather than his saints. So, I made an appointment to see Paul Niehans, the pioneer developer of cell therapy, or cellular therapy as he called it, in his clinic in Switzerland. He was, as a rule, available to physicians interested in his work.

I remember my visit as a unique experience. I was 44, and Niehans, in his 60's, was already the established *grand patron* of cell therapy. He was a tall, commanding man and addressed me as if I were a student. Niehans was a descendant, albeit illegitimate, of Frederick III of Prussia, and he had an imperial manner about him, dismissing with a slight frown and a tilt of the head even the slightest hint of an objection.

I did not in fact receive a satisfactory answer to the two questions I had in mind: did the cell injections really act as permanent implants, and could they really cure diabetes (the sweet diabetes or *mellitus*, characterized by high levels of sugar in the blood and urine)?

I fully agreed with Niehans that there was a cell organotropy, meaning that the injected cells act preferentially on their corresponding organs in the receiver organism. He theorized that live injected cells migrated to the corresponding organ of the host organism if this organ was in need of them, but this seemed doubtful to me. What seemed more likely (and this has since been partly confirmed in several experiments) was that the cells, once injected, released the vital *substances* they contained, and these substances gradually migrated to the site where their action was required. (Effects of cell therapy are latent; sometimes they are not observed until 12 to 14 weeks after injection.)

For the same reason, it was difficult for me to believe in the possibility of a cure for diabetes with cell injections. One of the major direct causes of diabetes is the malfunction of the islets of Langerhans, pancreatic cells that produce insulin. If live pancreatic cells were injected and had a chance to survive and function, a cure, at least partial, could theoretically be possible. But since they do not survive, there can be no possibility of cure. At best, temporary relief can be expected.

I saw Niehans extracting live cells from animals and treating patients at his famous clinic of La Prairie. I realized he was not an experimentalist but a superb clinician and diagnostician, who had developed his technique from experience (sometimes on himself) and after observing hundreds and thousands of favorable results achieved with cell therapy.

As I was working in Paris, he suggested that I get in touch with Dr. René Basile Henry, who is now France's foremost cell therapist. I later worked with Henry, a dedicated, rigorous physician, who introduced the use of lyophilized cells to France but who prefers for most cases to use fresh cells collected from animals raised at the farm operated for his clinic.

The advantage of freeze-dried cells is that dosages can be established more precisely and, of course, that the cells can be conserved. Most of the physicians who practice cell therapy, including myself, have found that the activity of freeze-dried cells is very close to that of fresh cells, unlike embryos, where the difference between freeze-dried and fresh is marked. At most, we can say that the duration of the biologic impulse given by freeze-dried cells is slightly lower than that of fresh cells.

The freeze-dried cells are obtained from a cell lyophilization plant founded by Niehans in Heidelberg. Since their widespread use began about 20 years ago, not a single case of infection has been reported.

In my practice, I have administered several thousand cell injections, without a single serious complication. There are very rare allergic reactions, but these can easily be overcome. When using fresh cells, absolute bacteriologic and serologic control of the donor animals must be exerted, and this requires an efficient laboratory setup and well-trained technicians to perform tests rapidly — as the injections must be made within minutes after the animal is killed. Health of living animals, of course, is also controlled.

Of course there were some accidents in the early days of cell therapy. Such accidents can occur with any kind of therapy, and when it comes to drugs, it is well known that the more effective the drug, the more severe are the potential side effects.

With cell therapy, accidents can occur as a result of allergies that have not been identified, or also when treatment is administered to heavily intoxicated or drug-addicted persons. With proper diagnosis these dangers can be avoided.

Indications for cell therapy must also be carefully examined. In my practice I find that on the average, 15 to 20 percent of the patients should not have cell injections, mostly because they suffer from inflammatory or infectious diseases. Drug addiction is another counterindication, and disturbances due to withdrawal symptoms are highly accentuated.

One aspect of cell therapy must be made very clear, for it is essential: The organotropic effect I have mentioned earlier cannot be reduced simply to a hormonal action, similar to that resulting from the injection of a synthetic hormone. Cell injections give completely different results. There is a primary effect, taking place within hours of the injection, that can be similar to that achieved with hormone injections and which indeed is due to the small doses of hormones contained in the ground-up cells. Much more important is the prolonged secondary effect, due to the stimulating influence the young cells have on the organ concerned in the injection. Many patients feel a surge of energy at first. This lasts a day or two and then passes, as the body's cells start to act on their own.

In this secondary effect, cell injections act in the opposite way from hormone injections. A continued administration of synthetic hormones or of hormones extracted from animal tissues can lead to a decreased function of the glands of the patient. The work that the glands should do is done by the needle, and there is a glandular disuse and "laziness." Cells, on the contrary, contain substances that activate the receiver's own organs and glands.

Experiments with animals have confirmed this. If injected cells are marked with a radioactive isotope, a study of the host organism with a Geiger counter shows an increased density of isotopes at the level of the homologous organ — that density corresponds to the injected cells. It has also been shown that mitosis (cell division) in the organ concerned with a particular cell injection is increased. This indicates that activating substances migrate to their new site of action.

Much research is still needed to elucidate the mechanism of this action, and this is not easy, because cells contain hormones, vitamins, and nucleic acids, as well as other organic elements in which some of these substances are concentrated. There may be hundreds of factors that have synergetic value, and it is presumptuous to think that if a few factors are isolated and even synthesized, the use of these synthetic substances, to the exclusion of others not yet known, will achieve the same results.

I grant that the mode of action of cell therapy has not been explained from A to Z. But many facts that correspond to the positive results obtained by cell therapy are known: the existence of organ-specificity from one species to another, the revitalizing effect of embryonic tissues upon old cells, the existence of organ-specific growth factors (trephones), and the existence of organ-specific growth inhibiting factors (chalones). How many drugs have been, and still are, used without one tenth of their mode of action or their side effects being known!

Arguments Against Cell Therapy

Some objection has been made to cell therapy on the grounds that it is dangerous. It can be dangerous, as can any therapy when it is attempted by an incompetent physician who does not take the whole organism into consideration when undertaking his treatment. By the same logic, a glass of water administered at the wrong time can be harmful.

After the first successful treatments with cell therapy were achieved by Niehans and his followers, many overenthusiastic, sometimes incompetent, sometimes profit-hungry physicians attempted to use the method without having sufficient knowledge of it and without control. Since then, several organizations have been formed in Europe to control cell therapy.

Cell therapy has been used also for the treatment of specific diseases. Professor F. Schmid, of Heidelberg, a respected German physician, has associated cell and other therapies to treat mongolism, a congenital, incurable disease characterized by a face with slanting eyes, a broad, short skull, broad hands, and short fingers. Mongolism is associated with severe mental retardation, and many of the children affected with it are institutionalized. Professor Schmid did not cure mongolism, but he has found that cell therapy could bring about considerable improvement. Out of the 380 cases he has treated, not one had to be institutionalized. In most of the children, there was an improvement of mental faculties, and many of them were able to attend school with normal children.

For the treatment, Professor Schmid used fetal brain cells as well as other cells chosen according to the specific deficiencies encountered in each case.

Recently physicians at the University of Wisconsin have found cell therapy to be effective for the treatment of congenital thymus dysfunction, which reflects itself in the total absence of immunologic defenses in a child. But all physicians who have had an extensive experience with it agree that it is particularly effective when used, in association with other therapies, against fatigue and troubles associated with aging.

If a physical examination, laboratory tests, and the history of a patient indicate that there is a weakening of an organ, appropriate cells can be chosen from a spectrum of over 60 cell types (all available in freeze-dried form). Three to four types of cells can be used simultaneously. Placenta and mesenchyme cells (embryonic tissues that will give rise to such structures as connective tissues, blood, bone, and cartilage) can be given for overall improvement, and other cells — hypothalamus, pancreas, liver — can be added to treat specific deficiencies of these organs. Testis cells can be used in almost every case after the age of 35 to 40 to maintain or improve male sexual function. In women, ovarian cells are used for the same purpose before menopause; after the ovaries have ceased functioning completely, there is no sense in administering ovarian cells, for they have nothing upon which to exercise an organotropic effect.

But it should not be said that cell therapy rejuvenates. It does not. Nothing does, and I think that the most likely means of rejuvenation would be in the realm of physics rather than medicine: to make time run backward. Let us be realistic, and see what cell therapy can do.

Applications of Cell Therapy

We have seen earlier that aging is not a uniform process. It is a degenerative disease that manifests itself in the organism's weakest links. Death is the breakage of *the* weakest link.

A physician concerned with revitalization must first find out what the weak links are and then do his utmost to strengthen them. Cell therapy is only one of the means to do this. It is, with embryotherapy, a medical act that goes beyond the maintenance of a healthy way of life by following some simple rules. Cell therapy is, for the time being, unfortunately reserved to a privileged few. I can only hope that this will not always be the case. (In Germany, certain forms of cell therapy are now covered by Social Security.)

It is an error, in my opinion, to consider the cell therapist as a specialist. Cell therapy is part of general medicine and should be integrated into it. It is true, of course, that a doctor using cell therapy must be thoroughly familiar with it. You do not prescribe cells as you prescribe aspirin.

The first thing is to determine the weak links and then to strengthen these, and also to strengthen those links which are known to be particularly important, and to strengthen, as much as possible, the whole chain.

Placenta cells are almost invariably given. These are the tissues that support and activate the development of the fetus. The effect is generalized, comparable to, but much greater and more long lasting than, the absorption of chicken embryos. Hypothalamus cells are usually used also, for the hypothalamus controls neurovegetative activity and influences the pituitary, which is said to be the conductor of the endocrine orchestra. Pituitary cells themselves should be used with particular caution in cases of pituitary insufficiency and never if there is an overproduction of pituitary hormones.

For men, I almost always administer testicular cells (these, of course, are taken from young animals and not from embryos). The sex glands are one of the most common weak links, and impotence is the chief complaint of people who seek revitalization.

But you do *not* treat impotence with cells. In a vast majority of cases, impotence originates in the mind, and it is there that the real treatment begins. The addition of cells is important because people who are impotent have not given their sexual glands all of the exercise, so to speak, that they deserve. Specific revitalizing action on these glands is helpful if the therapist succeeds in unblocking the mechanism that has caused impotence. I have treated countless cases of impotence, but not a single one with cells alone.

Perhaps the most spectacular results I have obtained were with an English patient, in his early 50's, who was suffering from secondary impotence resulting from a well-hidden feeling of guilt. It took him several weeks to realize and admit this guilt. Toward the end of the treatment, he received placenta cells as well as testicular cells.

He had a girlfriend, and shortly after the treatment, he informed me that performance was more than satisfactory. Then, a few months later, he wrote me that he was in trouble. It seems that another young lady he was courting showed some reluctance at the last moment (that was his version, anyway) and that he forced his way past her objections. Now, he said, he had been charged with rape! In fact, he was convicted and even served a prison sentence (for which, in spite of the successful treatment, I do not feel responsible; perhaps I helped restore a failing function, but I could not foresee the way in which it would be utilized).

Cell treatment, incidentally, is not effective in the treatment of homosexuality, even if a homosexual wants to be treated. Niehans believed it was, and one of his colleagues undertook an experiment involving some 50 homosexuals who were willing to try. Only one of the 50 reversed. Most of the others benefited from an increased sexual urge, but it was still aimed in the same direction.

Cell treatment *can* help relieve some sexual problems, notably infertility. A few cases have been reported of the treatment of oligospermia (low sperm count) with testicle injections along with other treatment, notably vitamin E.

For women, the equivalent, as I have mentioned earlier, is the injection of ovary cells. In conjunction with placenta cells, this can be very effective against troubles related to menopause. Cell treatment can help retard the onset of menopause by several years, as described in Chapter 18.

In the treatment of fatigue — not necessarily associated with aging — several types of cells, injected at the same time, usually give the best results: placenta, hypothalamus, testicles, liver, spleen, the selection of cells to be injected depending on the results of the prediagnostic tests. In the treatment of fatigue in men, testicular cells seem to be particularly effective. A series of clinical tests was conducted by the French physician Philippe Janson, who selected 25 subjects of the same age, similar occupations, and time schedules, and no specific organic disease but easy fatigability (both physical and mental). The experiment was done in three stages: a week of observation without treatment; four weeks of placebo treatment (injection of distilled water every other day); then treatment with one injection of ly-ophilized testicular cells. The patients did not know, at any time, what treatment they were receiving. Five parameters were observed throughout the test, with the following results:

During the first week, no change.

During the second period of four weeks, transitory improvements attributable to the placebo (suggestion) effect. Cell therapy, like almost any other therapy, evidently has a placebo effect.

Two to four weeks after the actual cell treatment, Dr. Janson noted a general feeling of increased vitality and well-being reported by 23 out of the 25 subjects. There was no change in pulse or arterial tension; a decrease of cholesterol, both total and circulating (perhaps attributable to increased activity); an increase in physical work capacity; and an increase of mental faculties in 25 percent of the cases, reflected by a decreased number of errors and more rapid performance in mental tests.

Results are even more remarkable in treating general loss of vitality and in delaying the gradual onset of degenerative diseases that are characteristic of aging. Many of the links in the organism are weakened, and the aging person is increasingly vulnerable to stresses he could cope with when younger.

It is in this area that the revitalizing effects of cell therapy are most obviously beneficial, whether fresh or freeze-dried cells are used.

But even in this preferential indication, it must not be forgotten that cell therapy is not a panacea, and it should not be the only means used toward the well-being and the restoration of the vitality of an aging person. It is part of a multitherapeutic approach, only one weapon, although a powerful one, in the modern arsenal of medicine.

Part V:
A Revitalized You

21. New Horizons, New Attitudes

If you drop a ring into the sea, your chances of finding it are very small indeed. But there *is* a chance, however infinitesimal, that you can find it, just as there is a chance that a coin you flip in the air will land on its edge, or that a number will come up a hundred straight times on the roulette wheel.

Almost anything that we lose can be regained. Sometimes it may be very difficult to get back, but few things are a total, irretrievable loss. Death, so far as we know, is one of them. Time is another. You cannot get time back. It is life.

Every hour that is lost, or badly filled, or miserably spent is permanently placed on the negative side of life. And you are the sum total of the hours you have lived. You exist only in relation to time. If all the hours you lived were to be miserable, painful, and devoid of joy and hope, life wouldn't have much point, but if you measured your life span not in terms of years expired but in terms of active, full, good hours passed, your life span would seem very short indeed. It would be enough merely to add some good hours and subtract bad ones in order to prolong it. This simple, evident, but usually overlooked, arithmetic is accessible to everyone. However, in spending our precious time, most of us, whatever our sex, age, job, or tax bracket, forget our most important asset: ourselves.

You are careful about damage that may occur to your house; you follow with some concern the ups and downs of any stock investment you may have, but you waste *yourself*, although you, a human being, may well be the most extraordinary, efficient, resistant achievement in the universe. This is criminal waste. You should take full advantage of what you are, but you should not be wasted, abused, or damaged, willfully or by neglect, either by yourself or by others.

No one is in a better position than you are to watch over yourself. True, when the need comes and something really goes wrong, experts are available to help. But when this help is required, it means that damage is already done and that it will be, at least to some extent, reflected in loss of vitality.

The trouble is that many of the signs of premature aging are taken for granted. We see them around us, they appear gradually, and we accept them as our lot. A most alarming fact is that the telltale signs of premature aging are appearing increasingly early, even in people in their 30's. At 40, many men look 50 and act as if they were 60. Women, more than men, resort to makeup and occasional plastic surgery to keep the appearance of youth, but the appearance, however important, is not the only element of youth.

In order to preserve you, your most important asset, you should, now and then, establish a balance sheet. It will not be checked by the IRS, and it should be frank and unbiased. It is something like a checklist you may make when purchasing a second-hand car. You are the one who will examine it and act upon its suggestions. I suggest you put it in the form of questions, and then write down the positive or negative answers. Ask yourself, for example, the following questions.

Are you chronically fatigued or frequently fatigued without any apparent reason?

Have you lost your appetite, lost the enjoyment of eating a good meal?

Have you weight problems? Are you either overweight or underweight to the point that you feel this problem to be a handicap?

Do you find it difficult to remember even important things? Try to determine whether the memory problem has been increasing.

Do you need a few drinks as a pick-me-up in the afternoon? I don't mean that you like to take a drink or two and enjoy it. I mean that you frequently feel toward the end of the day that you really *need* a drink, and if you don't have one, you become somewhat jittery about it.

Have you lost the urge for physical exertion or exercise? This question is particularly relevant if you do a sedentary type of work. The need for exercise should never disappear, although, of course, it is not the same at 30 as it is at 70.

Do you sleep well, or are you dependent upon sleeping pills?

Are you addicted to any kind of pill? Of course this does not include the taking of pills or injections for the treatment of a specific disease. It means the frequent, routine use of medicines, which is one of the most common forms of addiction nowadays.

Has your sex life become unsatisfactory? This can manifest itself in many ways, as we have seen earlier. Broadly speaking, have you either lost the ability to perform although the desire remains, or lost the desire, or libido? The second, more often than not, is a result of the first: you haven't been able to enjoy sexual relations as much as you used to, and you have persuaded yourself that you're not interested any more.

Have your bowels become lazy? Have you the feeling that abdominal muscles are loose and useless?

Do you feel you are getting out of touch, that you cannot keep up with your friends, that your life is limited to survival be-

tween work at the office or factory and collapse at home, where
you have barely the time to recover before the alarm clock jolts
you up for the following day's work?

Do you feel that you have lost your enthusiasm, that you have
less capacity for joy?

As a woman, are you overwhelmed with housework, overly
demanding of yourself to the most minute detail, and lacking
interest (or too tired) to do anything else?

These questions are the kind one forgets to ask oneself.
Civilized man has forgotten that premature aging is not inevitable and that one should not submit to it without question and
without rebellion. Old age must not be equated with senility.

Revitalization is a struggle against this premature aging, and
it can be an effective one. But before any struggle, one must
know its object, the means, and the goals that can be achieved.

This is vitally important, because our way of life is increasingly conducive to loss of vitality. We cannot really expect that
the stresses under which we have to live and function will disappear as if by magic. We cannot expect that our environment
will improve rapidly; we will be doing well enough if we keep it
from getting worse. We realize also that man's pace of life has
quickened and is still accelerating.

In the face of this, we must not give in. The public must
expect more than an indulgent smile, a pill, and a shrug of the
shoulder with the comment that "this is what you must expect."

If you realize that you are excessively fatigued, that you cannot sleep without a pill, that your sex life brings you no joy, you
must rebel. You must expect, and demand, more than you are
getting. If the public begins to expect more, to claim the full
benefits of the research and education it has, in the final
analysis, made possible through the taxes it pays, more doctors
will realize the shortcomings of modern medicine, and they will
search in the present and in the past for what has been lost,
neglected, or abandoned. They will seriously examine the
therapies that have been helping millions and will not reject or
ignore them simply because these therapies have not been developed in their time and under their particular national flag.

This is already beginning to happen.

In my practice I have had many doctors as patients. I have seen that many of the therapeutic methods I have used (although not invented) are increasingly applied by those doctors to their own patients. I am seeing on a larger scale what happened to a physician like my friend and colleague at Renaissance, Dr. William Goldwag, who was at first dubious about, then curious about, then intensely interested in certain treatments ignored in his country but widely practiced in others. This is happening, but it is happening too slowly.

I started this book by telling you that after 40 years of medical practice, I am dissatisfied. I am, because we could have progressed much more rapidly had we not been sidetracked by some of our prejudices and also by our own spectacular and heady achievements in the fields of medicine and biology. But I am also encouraged and somewhat relieved because, however belatedly, we are turning away from some of these prejudices, and, in terms of medicine, we are examining and beginning to make use of traditional, empirical knowledge we had long decided to ignore because we couldn't give it a formula.

New Horizons in Science

I see cell therapy, still controversial and once laughed at, being studied and put to use in several European countries, and achieving results not only in revitalization therapy but also in the treatment of such diseases as mongolism. Yet, cell therapy has not yet been the object of a single serious study in the United States.

I have seen embryotherapy tested in several European medical research centers and its efficacy discussed and demonstrated at the French Academy of Sciences. But embryotherapy has still not been studied in the United States.

However, I do see interest in treatments such as those developed by the Rumanian, Dr. Anna Aslan, who has achieved interesting results with a drug called gerovital, containing procaine (or Novocaine) and some additives. A dozen years ago when she first started speaking of her work, the reaction in the West was ironical derision. Since then it has been realized that the chemical structure of procaine is similar to that of para-aminobenzoic acid (PABA), a vitamin of the B complex, and that Dr. Aslan was neither a fool nor a charlatan.

I personally do not administer or prescribe Novocaine, as I believe that similar or better results can be achieved by natural biological means, without the unfavorable side effect which every synthetic product could possibly provoke.

It has long been established that all bodies in our universe that have a temperature above absolute zero emit electromagnetic radiation, and radiometry has made it possible to measure this radiation. We know not only that our organism has very specific electromagnetic fields but that these can be influenced by other fields. We know this influence can be beneficial but also that it can be harmful, even deadly. The existence of these fields in every living being from plants to man has been shown, notably in the work of Dr. Saxton Burr of Yale, who refers to them as "life fields."

How our electromagnetic fields are influenced by, and interact with, surrounding fields is the subject of research in many countries. It has been observed that birds collapse even in moderate microwave fields, that there is a change in the production of chicken eggs, that brain waves are altered, that vegetation growth is slowed down or completely interrupted. There is an effect on the rate of flow of liquids (such as blood) in tubes of small diameter. High fields provoke a loss of myelin, a substance covering nerve fibers, and cause cell destruction. There have been several accidental deaths, in the United States and elsewhere, from exposure to electromagnetic fields generated by large radars, such as are used in radio astronomy.

Interference with natural electromagnetic fields has been associated with behavioral changes. This is not surprising, and there is no doubt that these fields can contribute, to an extent that is still unknown, to the stress we are subjected to in our self-made environment, and to loss of vitality.

The live embryo has its specific electromagnetic field, different from that of a fresh, nonincubated egg, which has, in turn, a field different from that of a boiled egg or an omelet. When you swallow a live incubated egg, its electromagnetic field — for a time, however short — exists within you. We know also that fields in your organism interact with outside fields and with fields introduced into it. How they interact, we do not know. Soviet researchers have announced recently that they have found that cells communicate between themselves with the help of such fields, and this communication can take place even if the cells are separated by a membrane, such as the gastrointestinal lining.

We know also that when chick embryo juice is introduced into a chicken cell culture, this culture continues multiplying. Alexis Carrel's well-known experiment has demonstrated that if this juice is not introduced, the cells do not continue multiplying and die. I do not say that Carrel's hypothetic trephones can be identified with electromagnetic fields; we don't know yet, but this seems to be a reasonable hypothesis. It could account for the effects of embryotherapy and of cell therapy.

In cell therapy, as in embryotherapy, there is a transmission of revitalizing elements. Their action cannot be explained entirely in terms of biochemistry. Isn't it conceivable that electromagnetic fields hold the answer, or at least part of it?

Earlier, we described how psychic phenomena are now coming to the forefront of medical research. I find this simple recognition of the body-mind unit the single most encouraging and promising trend in today's medicine. We are becoming more open-minded, we no longer reject dogmatically something that we haven't learned in medical school, that cannot be entirely explained, or that does not have a formula. It is significant that an American pharamaceutical company has already started serious research into the therapeutic potential of what may one day be referred to as "psychic medicine," even though the company is aware that its own research may lead to an abrupt decrease in the use of psychotropic drugs, which have represented an increasing source of income to it since their discovery some 20 years ago.

New Attitudes Toward Aging

We are also becoming more open-minded with regard to our prejudices as a youth-oriented society. Some of these prejudices still exist, of course, and will for years to come.

For centuries, mankind has relied on the young — the very young — for productivity and procreation. But since the turn of the century, the proportion of the population over 65 has approximately doubled in many industrial countries, such as the United States, Great Britain, Germany, and France. The attitudes of society have not followed this trend. We have remained youth-oriented, and we have not adapted to the fact that the population has grown not only larger but older. This maladaption is evident in two fields of activity traditionally attributed to youth: work and sexual activity. There is no need to expand on either — we all know of the employer's preference for the young executive and society's derisive attitude toward the fact that older people can have an active sexual life.

It is true that the highest and best productivity in some intellectual and artistic fields comes in early life. This is true of physics, chemistry, psychology, painting, literature, mathematics, and even more so of lyric poetry. But most researchers now agree that chronologic age alone is an uncertain indicator of physical or intellectual ability.

A study by Canadian science writer David Spurgeon shows that mental deterioration and deterioration of performance are, very often, not the result of the aging process itself, but the result of the social pressures in our society, and a fear of aging.

Those people who rise above this fear and who are not touched by social pressures of the youth-oriented society escape the fate that is too often accepted without question. Spurgeon points out, for instance, that an analysis of the productivity of Thomas A. Edison shows a peak around age 35, a decline at 47 and 48, a secondary peak around 57, and a third between 70 and 75, brought on by the stimulus of the World War I.

Some people, in their older years, turn to new careers. General Eisenhower and General de Gaulle, for example, both abandoned the military to turn to politics. Continued interest in one's area of interest and preference, added to the experience of age, shows that creativity can remain vigorous into older years. Such examples as Picasso, Matisse, and Casals are well known because these were famous people. Others, away from the limelight, are countless, not only in artistic and intellectual fields, but in all fields, including medicine, carpentry, and watchmaking.

Another false problem is the "old worker problem case." Such cases have been used to justify some managerial attitudes, but many of these cases, when examined closely, turn out to be of people who became a problem long before they became older workers. As they approach a retirable age, the urge to solve the problem increases, and they become the "older worker problem case," neatly fitting into an accepted pattern.

Yet another misconception is that expressed by the saying that "you can't teach an old dog new tricks." Most psychologists and gerontologists now agree that one does not grow too old to learn. Dr. Wilder Penfield, the well-known Canadian neurosurgeon and the author of *The Second Career*, has suggested that even an octogenarian can learn if sufficiently motivated. The senior citizen should not hide behind the too-easy excuse of old age or senescence as a reason for not leading an active life.

Of course, with increasing age, there may be less muscular strength, less intense emotional drive. But skills tend to improve with long practice, and there is a better defined purpose of living with increased maturation.

We are beginning to accept this, and youth-oriented prejudices may be gradually disappearing. But here, too, the process is slow.

Still, we must not give up. We have seen that the life span of man in many industrial countries has started to decline. It is possible and even probable that the next generation, or the one after that, will benefit fully from the explosion of medical science against aging that we are entitled to expect. In the meanwhile, each of us can take advantage of what is already known to make his life better, fuller, and longer.

22. Your Potential for Staying Young

I am not an apostle for any particular type of therapy. I know there is no elixir of youth to drink, no Shangri-La to shelter us. The multitherapeutic approach to revitalization offers a number of small solutions, suggests a number of slight changes. None of these, by itself, is overly important. But add them up, and you will find that surprising results can be achieved.

The hints I have given you are the results of my experience. I don't think that any one of them is too unpleasant, cumbersome, or time-consuming. All of us are aware of the importance of the food we eat, but some aspects of nutrition are generally overlooked. We have seen that one of the most important ones is our need for raw food, live elements that have a revitalizing action, and whose absence is harmful.

All of us know, also, that weight is an important factor. There is no need to become a professional weight-watcher, but do not let weight build up gradually and unnoticed until you are severely overweight. Overweight is always associated with loss of vitality.

Don't forget that with nutrition, as with anything else, an occasional change of pace is beneficial. A fruit or vegetable cure, an occasional fast, help you get rid of accumulated toxins. When I say fast, I do not mean starvation. It is enough to omit one particular type of food, such as meat or fat, for a few days and to avoid alcoholic beverages during the same period. I am not a teetotaler, but an occasional break in the drinking habit is to be recommended, if only to make sure, now and then, that you aren't addicted to the point of being unable to stop.

Just as your digestive system needs an occasional change, so do you. The Sabbath day of rest, like the fast, makes good sense. Try to make sure that the periodic break you give yourself is really a complete break from routine and from your surroundings. If you are a city dweller, leave the city and breathe some fresh air. Don't spend a week in town reading, going to the movies or to restaurants. The five-day week gives you frequent opportunities for such minor changes of pace on weekends.

In your leisure time, avoid the shock element — you probably have enough of that in your daily life, on television, and in the newspapers. Seek beauty, which inevitably weighs on the positive side.

If you have hobbies, try to spend some time on those that represent an activity entirely different from your work routine. An engineer shouldn't spend his weekends on the upkeep and maintenance of toy trains, and an accountant might find something else to do besides collecting stamps, though it might be a good change for a busy housewife.

Husband and wife must team up to break the monotony of everyday life. An unexpected outing, champagne and caviar by the fireplace, erotic games, reversal of usual roles — there are a thousand ways, which I leave to your imagination.

When you are at home, or in the country, avoid some of the constraints imposed by society. Be natural: take your shoes off, for instance. Giving some freedom to your feet is a much better way to keep away infection than letting them macerate in your shoes after covering them with a deodorant or antiperspirant powder.

I am not a barefoot doctor or a nudist, but I do recommend that the body be freed, and not only during sleep, from buttons, zippers, belts, collars, socks, garters, and shoes. Even in town, you can occasionally give your body the luxury of a breath of fresh air. After a rain, the air is cleaned of dust and smoke; open your window and stand in front of it, undressed, and take a few deep breaths. (If there are neighbors across the street, don't forget to draw the curtains or turn out the lights — there's no sense in provocation.)

Avoid, as much as possible, the habit of taking medicine regularly. The addiction to sleeping pills can usually be prevented, either by learning to relax or by using, when needed, natural elements such as honey, chamomile, or orange flower infusions. One of the physicians I have treated told me, not long before this writing, that he has tried this treatment on twenty of his patients who were either habituated to sleeping pills or who could not sleep well in spite of sleeping pills. He was delighted to have found that all responded, either to chamomile or to orange flowers, and that in all cases but one, the use of sleeping pills was discontinued.

You can also contribute to a fuller, richer, and healthier life by maintaining an active interest in sex, by not letting your sex life become a Saturday night habit, by trying variants and sex games, and, above all, by never considering sex as an obligation to be fulfilled. Both partners should understand and agree to this; sex is a *pacte à deux*.

With sex, as with anything else, an occasional fast is beneficial. If you feel you are losing interest in sex, that it is becoming a routine, break the habit. Make the decision, with your spouse or partner, to abstain for a given time, say a week, or whatever period would represent, in your case, unusually long abstinence. During that time, there should be nothing to stop you from thinking about sex, or talking about it, from reading Casanova or dancing the tango, but make it a point not to break the resolution while preparing yourself for the banquet ahead.

Throughout my personal life and my professional life, I have, so to speak, kept score: this goes in red and to the left of the balance sheet, this goes to the right, in black. Many of the entries may seem so unimportant that one neglects to make the small effort required to transfer the item from the negative to the positive side. By forgetting to do it for a long enough time, the balance eventually tips the wrong way.

If you have sinned against yourself by omission, it is not too late to repent. The hints I have given in this book are examples of what can be done, and there are many other examples that you can easily discover for yourself, once you are conscious of the importance of a positive balance.

Do not let life pass by and your surroundings dominate you. Use your vitality to live fully, and do not forget to replenish your vitality supply at the slightest opportunity, for there is no service station on your way to fill up the tank.

The closest to this, and undoubtedly the highest grade of fuel available, is joy. But remember, it's not a usual kind of commodity, for the best way to receive it is to give it away.

The revitalizing potential of joy is tremendous. I, and others, have witnessed the complete metamorphosis of people who had given up, grown old under great stress. Joy, hope, and enthusiasm have acted as if they were the closest things to a fountain of youth.

Joy is the light that illuminates the way ahead.

Selected Readings

Backle, B. 1963. "Experimental Evaluation of Work Capacity as Related to Chronological and Physiological Ageing," Civil Aeronautics Research Institute, FAA. Oklahoma City, Okla.: CARI Report (September), pp. 63–78.

Barber, Theodore, et al., (eds.). 1970. *Biofeedback and Self-Control.* Chicago: Aldine-Atherton.

———, et al. (eds.). 1971. *Biofeedback and Self-Control Reader.* Chicago: Aldine-Atherton.

Barnett, S. A. 1967. "Rats," *Scientific American,* 216: 78–85.

Barraclough, C. A. 1966. "Modifications in the Central Nervous System Regulation of Reproduction after Exposure of Prepubertal Rats to Steroid Hormone," *Recent Progress in Hormone Research,* 22: 503–528.

Beach, F. A. (ed.). 1965. *Sex and Behavior.* New York: Wiley.

Beer, Alan E., and Rupert E. Billingham. 1974. "The Embryo as a Transplant," *Scientific American*, 230: 36–46.

Benjamin, H. 1945. "Eugen Steinach, 1861–1944: A Life of Research," *Science Monthly*, 61: 427–442.

Benson, Herbert and D. Shapiro, B. Tursky and G. Schwartz. 1971. "Decreased Systolic Blood Pressure Through Operant Conditioning Techniques in Patients with Essential Hypertension," *Science*, 173: 740–742.

Bernard, Claude. 1927. *An Introduction to the Study of Experimental Medicine.* Trans., Harry Copley Greene. New York: Macmillan.

———. 1974. *Lectures on the Phenomena of Life Common to Animals and Plants.* Trans., Habel E. Hoff, Roger Guillemin, and Lucienne Guillemin. Springfield, Ill.: American Lecture Series.

Best, C. H., and N. B. Taylor. 1961. *The Physiological Basis of Medical Practice.* Baltimore: Williams and Wilkins.

Bjorksten, John. 1962. "Aging: Present Status of Our Chemical Knowledge," *Journal of the American Geriatric Society*, 10: 125–139.

———. 1963. "Aging, Primary Mechanism," *Gerontologia*, 8:179–192.

Bodenstein, Dietrich, and Karl Maramorosch, F. Engelman, et al. 1960. "Aspects of Insect Endocrinology," *Annals of the New York Academy of Sciences*, 89: 487–571.

Bordet, Jules. 1898. *"Sur l'agglutination et la dissolution des globules rouges par le serum d'animax injectes de sang defibrine,"* *Annales de l'Institut Pasteur.*

Bowen, Humphrey J. M. 1966. *Trace Elements in Biochemistry.* London: Academic Press.

Brekhman, I. I. 1967. "Panax Ginseng—I," *Medical & Science Service*, Vol. 4. Calcutta.

———. 1969. "New Substances of Plant Origin Which Increase Nonspecific Resistance." Reprinted from *Annual Review of Pharmacology*, 9: 419–430.

———, and I. V. Dardymov. "Pharmacological Investigation of Glycosides from Ginseng and Eleutherococcus." Published by The Institute of Biologically Active Substances, Siberian Branch of The Academy of Sciences, Vladivostok, U.S.S.R. Translation supplied by Pharmaton, Ltd., Lugano, Switzerland.

———, and M. A. Grinevich. "Method of Biological Standardization of Panax Ginseng by Its Antidiuretic Action." Published by The Institute of Biologically Active Substances, Siberian Branch of The Academy of Sciences, Vladivostok, U.S.S.R. Translation supplied by Pharmaton, Ltd., Lugano, Switzerland.

Breton, Guilloume. 1942. *Considerations sur l'étiopathogenie du mongolisme.* Paris: T.E.P.A.C.

Briggs, Michael H., and J. Brotherton. 1970. *Steroid Biochemistry and Pharmacology*. London, New York: Academic Press.

Bullough, William Sydney. 1967. *The Evolution of Differentiation*. London: Academic Press.

Burnet, Macfarlane. 1961. "The Mechanism of Immunity," *Scientific American*, 204: 58–67.

———. "The Thymus Gland," *Scientific American*, 207: 50–57.

Burr, Harold, S. 1973. *The Fields of Life: Our Links with the Universe*. New York: Ballantine Books, Inc.

Carrel, Alexis. 1924. "Leucocytic Trephones," *Journal of the American Medical Association*, 52: 255–258.

———. 1926. "Things That Doctors Do Not Know," in Paul Luttinger (ed.), *Cancer*. Vol. 4. New York: 1:16–21.

———. 1928. "The Mechanism of Senesence," *Bulletin of The New York Academy of Medicine*, 4: 1144–46.

———. 1935. *Man the Unknown*. New York and London: Harper & Brothers.

———, and Charles Augustus Lindberg. 1938. *The Culture of Organs*. New York: P. B. Hoeber.

———. 1938a. *Cancer et tréphones de Carrel*. Paris: E. Le François.

Cheney, Garnett. 1944. "Duodenal Ileus and Stasis," in Portis (ed.). *Diseases of the Digestive System*. Philadelphia: Portis, pp. 309–378.

———. 1950. *Medical Management of Gastrointestinal Disorders*. Chicago: Year Book Publishers.

Comfort, Alex. 1966. *Sex in Society*. Secaucus, N. J.: Citadel Press, Inc.

Corner, G. W. 1963. *Hormones in Human Reproduction*. New York: Atheneum.

Corners, George. 1973. *Rejuvenation: How Steinach Makes People Young*. New York: Seltzer.

Cutting, W. C. 1969. *Handbook of Pharmacology*. New York: Appleton-Century-Crofts.

Damreau, Frederic. 1964. *Therapeutic Uses of Yogurt; A Review of the Literature*. New York: International Yogurt Foundation.

Davies, David. 1973. "A Shangri-la in Ecuador," *New Scientist*, 57: 236–238.

Dovring, Folke. 1974. "Soybeans," *Scientific American*, 230: 14–22.

Dubos, René. 1965. *Man Adapting*. New Haven, Conn.: Yale University Press.

———, and Maya Pines. 1965. *Health and Disease. Life Science Library*. New York: Time, Inc.

———. 1968. *Men, Medicine and Environment*. New York: Frederick A. Praeger.

Ellis, John Marion, and James Presley. 1973. *Vitamin B6: The Doctor's Report.* New York: Harper & Row.

Engel, B. and R. Chism. 1967. "Operant Conditioning of Heart Rate Speeding," *Psychophysiology,* 3: 418–187.

————.1966. "Operant Conditioning of Heart Rate Slowing," *Psychophysiology,* 3:176–187.

Etkin, William (ed.). 1964. *Social Organization and Behavior Among Vertebrates.* Chicago: University of Chicago Press.

Fieser, L. F. 1955. "Steroids," *Scientific American,* 192: 52–60.

Filatov, Vladimir. 1943. *Tkanevaya terapiya (lechnie fiziologicheski mi stimulyatorami tkanevego proislchojdenya);* podredaktiey, B. I. Berlinera i Ya. M. Bruskina. [*Tissue Therapy: (Treatment Based on Physiological Stimulation of Tissues)*], B. I. Berliner and Ya. M. Breskina (eds.). Tashkent, USSR: GOSIDAT.

Franklin, Olga. 1964. *H3: An Account of the Work of Professor Anna Aslan with the H3 Drug as Preventive Treatment for the Signs and Symptoms of Old Age.* London: Arthur Barber.

Fredericks, Carlton, and Herman Goodman. 1973. *Low Blood Sugar and You.* New York: Grosset & Dunlap.

Friedrich, Rudolph. 1961. *Frontiers of Modern Medicine.* London: Collier-Macmillan, Ltd.

Gibbons, Euell. 1970. *Stalking the Wild Asparagus.* New York: David McKay Company.

Goodman, Herman. 1961. *Professor Doctor Anna Aslan: Her Work.* New York: Medical Lay Press.

Gray, C. M. (ed.). 1966. *Gray's Anatomy of the Human Body.* Philadelphia: Lea and Febiger.

Green, E., A. Green, and E. Walters. 1970. "Self-regulation of Internal States," in J. Rose (ed.). *Progress of Cybernetics: Proceedings of the International Congress of Cybernetics, London, 1969.* London: Gordon and Breach.

Griffon, Henri. 1958. "La deshydration des substances d'origine biologique animale ou végétale en vue de l'alimentation, la diététique, la thérapeutique." Paris: Private printing.

————, 1958. "Une machine à deshydrater les produits biologiques (deux types)." Paris: Private printing.

Haire, Norman. 1924. *Rejuvenation: The Work of Steinach, Voronoff and Others.* London: George Allen & Unwin, Ltd.

Hannon, Leslie. 1972. *The Second Chance: The Life and Work of Dr. Paul Niehans*. London, New York: Allen.

Harman, D. 1952. "Aging: A Theory Based on Free Radical and Radiation Chemistry," *Journal of Gerontology*, 11: 298–300.

Harms, Ernest. 1969. "Correspondence Between Eugen Steinach and Harry Benjamin," *Bulletin of the New York Academy of Medicine*, 45: 761–766.

Hayflick, Leonard. 1968. "Human Cells and Aging," *Scientific American*, 218: 32–37.

The Herbalist Almanac. 1970. Indianapolis, Ind.: Indiana Botanical Gardens.

Hollister, L. E. 1971. "Hunger and Appetite after Single Doses of Marihuana, Alcohol and Dextroamphetamine," *Clinical Pharmacology and Therapeutics*, 12: 44–49.

Jensen, W. A. 1962. *Botanical Histochemistry: Principles and Practice*. San Francisco: Freeman.

Kapleau, Philip. 1967. *The Three Pillars of Zen*. Boston: Beacon Press.

Kelsay, J. L. 1969. "A Compendium of Nutritional Status Studies and Dietary Evaluation Studies Conducted in the United States, 1957–1967," *Journal of Nutrition*, 99 (Supplement 1, Part 2): 123–166.

Kinsey, A. C., W. B. Pomeroy, and C. E. Martin. 1948. *Sexual Behavior in the Human Male*. Philadelphia: Saunders.

———, et al. 1953. *Sexual Behavior in the Human Female*. Philadelphia: Saunders.

Kodicek, Egon. 1956. "Metabolic Studies on Vitamin D," in Wolstonholme (ed.), *Bone Structure and Metabolism*. Boston: Little, Brown, and Company, pp. 161–174.

Lambert, Gilles. 1959. *The Conquest of Age: The Extraordinary Story of Dr. Paul Niehans*. New York: Rinehart and Company.

Lang, P. J. 1970. "Autonomic Control," *Psychology Today*, 4: 37–41.

Lansford, E. M., Jr., and William Shive. 1955. "Antimetabolites in the Study of the Biochemistry of Purines and Pyrimidines," in *Antimetabolites and Cancer*. Washington: American Association for the Advancement of Science, pp. 33–45.

Lawson-Wood, Denis, and Joyce Lawson-Wood. 1964. *Acupuncture Handbook*. Rustington, England: Health Science Press.

Leaf, Alexander. 1973. "Search for the Oldest People," *National Geographic*, 143: 93–119.

Lingbeck, Goswijn. 1908. *Zeewater als genee smiddel (Sabentane methode Quinton).* Amsterdam: F. van Rosson.

Lucas, Richard. 1969. *Nature's Medicines.* New York: Parker Publishing Company.

McCay, C. M. 1939. "Chemical Aspects of Ageing," in A. Cowdry (ed.)., *Problems of Ageing.* Baltimore: Johns Hopkins Press, pp. 572–623.

———. 1973. "'Notes on the History of Nutrition Research," F. Verzar (ed.). Bern: Hans Huber.

Marx, Henry. 1960. *"H3 in the Battle Against Old Age; A Dramatic New Use for Novocaine.* New York: Plenum Press.

Masters, William, and Virginia Johnson. 1966. *Human Sexual Response.* Boston: Little, Brown and Company.

———. 1970. *Human Sexual Inadequacy.* Boston: Little, Brown, and Company.

Mathé, Georges, Jean-Louis Amiel, and Leon Schwarzenberg. 1971. *Bone Marrow Transplantation and Leucocyte Transfusions.* Springfield, Ill.: Thomas.

———, and M. Tubiana (eds.). 1973. *The Natural History, Diagnosis and Treatment of Hodgkin's Disease.* Series Haematologica. Vol. 6. Copenhagen: Munksgaard.

Mayer, Jean. 1956. "Appetite and Obesity," *Scientific American,* 108: 30–36.

Medawar, P. B. 1957. "Skin Transplants," *Scientific American,* 196: 62–69.

Medical World News, "Biofeedback in Action," March 9, 1973, Vol. 14, p. 47.

Medvedev, M. A. (Zhores). 1966. *Protein Biosynthesis and Problems of Heredity, Development and Aging.* Edinburgh: Oliver and Boyd.

———. 1963. "The Effect of Ginseng on the Working Performance of Radio Operators," *Papers on the Study of Ginseng and Other Medicinal Plants of the Far East,* Issue 5, p. 237. Vladivostok, U.S.S.R.

———. 1970. *Molecular-Genetic Mechanisms of Development.* Trans., Basil Haigh. New York: Plenum Press.

Metchnikoff, Elie. 1910. *The Prolongation of Life: Optimistic Studies.* Trans., P. Chalmers Mitchell. New York: G. P. Putnam's Sons.

———, and Eugene Wollman. 1913. *Some Researches on Intestinal Disinfection with the* Bacillus bulgaricus *and* Glycobacter *peptolyticus in Symbiosis.* New York: American Institute of Pasteur.

Mick, Stephan S. 1975. "The Foreign Medical Graduate," *Scientific American,* 232: 14–21.

Miller, Neal. 1969. "Learning of Visceral and Glandular Responses," *Science*, 163: 434–445.

———, John Dollard, Leonard Doob, O. H. Mourer, Robert Sears, et al. 1971. *Frustration and Aggression*. New Haven, Conn.: Yale University Institute of Human Relations.

Morelle, Jean. 1957. *Traite de Biochimie Cutance*. Paris: Éditions Varia.

———. 1964. *Chimie et biochimie des lipides*. 3 vols. Paris: Éditions Varia.

Moscona, Aron. 1950. *Studies on the Anatomy and the Histology of the Pancreas in Snakes and Lizards*. Jerusalem: Jerusalem Press.

———. 1959. "Tissues from Dissociated Cells," *Scientific American*, 200: 132–139.

———. 1961. "How Cells Associate," *Scientific American*, 205: 142–160.

Moss, Louis. 1964. *Acupuncture and You; A New Approach to Treatment Based on the Ancient Method of Healing*. London: Elek Books.

Naranjo, Claudio. 1970. "Present Centeredness: Technique, Prescription and Ideal," in Joen Fagen and Irma Lee Sheperd (eds.). *Gestalt Therapy Now*. New York: Harper & Row.

Niehans, Paul. 1948. *Biological Treatment of Disease Organs in Human Beings and Animals*. Interlaken: O Schaefli.

———. 1957. *Einführung in die Zellular-Therapie; Vorlesung*. Bern: Hans Huber.

———. 1960. *Introduction to Cellular Therapy*. New York: Pageant Books.

———. 1961. "B-Cells on the Islets of Langerhans in the Fight against Pancreatic Diabetes Mellitus," *Third Report on the Present State of Research*. Bern: Hans Huber.

———. 1969. *The Cancer Problem*. Bern: Stäpeli et Cie.

Olmstead, James Montrose Duncan. 1946. *Charles Edouard Brown-Sequard, A 19th Century Neurologist and Endocrinologist*. Baltimore: Johns Hopkins Press.

Orentreich, Norman. 1959. "Autographs in Alopeias and Other Selected Dermatological Conditions," *Archives of the New York Academy of Science*, 83: 463–479.

Ornstein, Robert E. 1972. *The Psychology of Consciousness*. New York: The Viking Press.

Pauling, Linus. 1970. *Vitamin C and the Common Cold*. San Francisco: Freeman and Company.

Penfield, Wilder. 1947. "Psychical Seizures," in C. K. Drinker, et al. (eds.). *Psychiatric Research*. Cambridge, Mass., pp. 81–99.

————. 1952. "Memory Mechanisms," reproduced with additions in *American Medical Association Archives of Neurology and Psychiatry*. Vol. 67. Chicago, pp. 178–191.

————. 1963. "The Chinese People's Republic: A Physician's Observations," Horowitz Lectures. New York: Institute of Physical Medicine and Rehabilitation.

————. 1963. *The Second Career, with Other Essays and Addresses*. Boston: Little, Brown, and Company.

Pottenger, Francis M., Jr. 1946. "Effect of heat-processed foods and metabolized vitamin D milk on the dento-facial structures of experimental animals," *American Journal of Orthodontics and Oral Surgery*, 32: Section Oral Surgery, pp. 467–485.

Pratt, Viola Whitney. 1956. *Famous Doctors: Osler, Banting, Penfield*. Toronto: Clarke, Irwin and Company.

Present Knowledge in Nutrition. 1967. New York: The Nutrition Foundation, Inc.

Rammurt, Misha. 1959. *Fundamentals of Yoga*. New York: Julian Press.

Roels, Oswald. 1967. "Present Knowledge of Vitamin E," *Nutrition Reviews*. Vol. 25: 33–37.

Root, Waverley. 1975. "Taste Is Falling! Taste Is Falling!" *The New York Times Magazine* (February 16), p. 18.

Rose, Jeanne. 1972. *Herbs and Things; Jeanne Rose's Herbal*. New York: Grosset & Dunlap.

Saint-Exupéry, Antoine de. 1970. *Le Petit Prince*. Miller, J. (ed.). Boston: Houghton Mifflin Company.

Sargent, J., E. Green, and E. Walters. "Preliminary Report on the Use of Autogenic Feedback Techniques in the Treatment of Migraine and Tension Headaches." Unpublished manuscript, Menninger Foundation, Topeka, Kan. 1971.

Scicenkov, M. V. 1963. "The Effect of Liquid Extracts of the Ginseng and Eleutherococcus on Dark Adaptation and Visual Acuity," *Papers on the Study of Ginseng and Other Medicinal Plants of the Far East*, Issue 5, p. 241. Vladivostok, U.S.S.R.

Selye, Hans. October 6, 1947. "The Diseases of Adaptation with Main Emphasis upon Hypertension." The Ludwig Kast Lecture. Graduate Fortnight of the New York Academy of Medicine.

————. 1950. "The Physiology and Pathology of Stress," *Annual Report on Stress*, Vol. 1.

————. 1950a. "Historia de la endocrinologia," in *Tratado de Endocrinologia Clinica*. Vol. 1. Buenos Aires, pp. 15–56.

————. 1953. "The General Adaptation Syndrome in its Relationships to Neurology, Psychology, and Psychopathology," in *Contributions Toward Medical Psychology*. Vol. 1. New York: Weider, pp. 234–274.

————. 1956. *The Stress of Life*. New York: McGraw-Hill.

————. 1962. *Calciphylaxis*. Chicago: University of Chicago Press.

————. 1964. *From Dream to Discovery; On Being a Scientist*. New York: McGraw-Hill.

————. 1971. *Hormones and Resistance*. New York: Springer.

Shive, William, et al. 1950. "The Biochemistry of B Vitamins." American Chemical Society Monograph Series, #110. New York: Rheinholt Publishing Corporation.

Shute, Evan Vere. 1956. *Your Heart and Vitamin E*. New York: Devin-Adair Company.

Sidel, Victor, and Ruth Sidel. 1974. "The Delivery of Medical Care in China," *Scientific American*, 230: 19–27.

Sokolov, Raymond. 1975. "A Plant of Ill Repute," *Natural History*, 83: 70–71.

Spittle, C. R. 1971. "Atherosclerosis and Vitamin C," *Lancet*, 2:1280–1281.

Steinach, Eugen. 1920. "Verjungen durch experimentelle neubelung der alternden pubertäts drüse." Monograph. Berlin: J. Springer.

Still, Joseph William. 1958. *Science Education at the Crossroads: A View from the Laboratory*. Washington: Public Affairs Press.

Stillman, William B. 1935. "An Analytical Study of Invertase Soluble in Saturated Aqueous Ammonium Sulfate." Thesis. New York: Columbia University.

Stone, Irwin. 1972. *The Healing Factor; Vitamin C Against Disease*. New York: Grosset & Dunlap.

Stough, D. Bluford, III. 1973. "Current Trends in Hair Transplantation," *Archives of Otolaryngology*, 98: 370–372.

Tappel, A. L. 1963. "Vitamin E Deficiency in Rabbits," *Nutrition Reviews*, 21: 23.

————. 1967. "Where Old Age Begins," *Nutrition Today*, Vol. 2, #4 (December), pp. 2–7. Published by the Florida Citrus Commission.

————. 1968. "Will Antioxidant Nutrients Slow Aging Processes?" *Geriatrics*, 23: 97–105.

Taylor, Renee. 1966. *Hunza Health Secrets for Long Life and Happiness*. Englewood Cliffs, N.J.: Prentice-Hall, Inc.

Underwood, Eric John. 1956. *Trace Elements in Human and Animal Nutrition*. New York: Academic Press.

Voronoff, Serge. 1920. *Life: A Study of the Means of Restoring Vital Energy and Prolonging Life*. Trans., Evelyn Bostwick Voronoff. New York: E. P. Dutton & Co.

————. 1925. *Rejuvenation by Grafting*. Trans., Fred F. Imianitoff. London: George Allen & Unwin, Ltd.

————. 1926. *The Study of Old Age and My Method of Rejuvenation*. Trans., Fred F. Imianitoff. London: Gill Publishing Company.

————. 1928. *The Conquest of Life*. Trans., G. Gibier Rambaud. New York: Brentano.

————, and George Alexandiescu. *Testicular Grafting from Ape to Man; Operative Technique, Physiological Manifestations, Histological Evolution, Statistics*. Trans., T. C. Merrill. London: Brentano.

————. 1939. *Greffe des glandes endocrines: la méthode, la technique, les résultats*. Paris: G. Doin et Cie.

————. 1941. *From Cretin to Genius*. New York: Alliance Book Corporation.

————. 1943. *The Sources of Life*. Toronto: The Ryerson Press.

Walford, Roy Lee. 1969. "The Isoantigenic Systems of Human Leukocytes: Medical and Biological Significance," in *Series Haematologica*. Vol. 2:2. Copenhagen: Montesgaard.

Weiner, Michael A. 1972. *Earth Medicine—Earth Foods*. New York: Macmillan.

Weiss, Paul. 1939. *Principles of Development; A Text in Experimental Embryology*. New York: H. Holt and Company.

————. 1971. *Biomedical Excursions; A Biologist's Probings into Medicine*. New York: Hafner.

————. 1973. *The Science of Life; The Living System—A System for Living*. Mt. Kisco, New York: Futura.

Williams, Roger J. 1971. "How Can the Climate in Medical Education be Changed?" in D. J. Ingle (ed.). Vol. 14. *Perspectives in Biology and Medicine*, pp. 608–614.

Winter, Ruth. 1972. *A Consumer's Dictionary of Food Additives*. New York: Crown Publishing Company.

Wolf, Max, and Karl Ransberger. 1972. *Enzyme Therapy*. New York: Vantage Press.

World Health Organization. 1972. *World Health Statistics Report*, 25: 430–442.

Zo Bell, Claude E. 1946. *Marine Microbiology: A Monograph on Hydrobacteriology*. Waltham, Mass.: Chronica Botanica Company.

Index